Navigating the Maze During Treatment of Adult Survivors of Child Psychological Abuse: Severe Parental Alienation

A Comprehensive Resource Guide for Mental Health Practitioners, Offering Insights, Strategies and Risk Mitigation from a PhD Thesis on the Challenges Faced by Practitioners Treating Adult Child Survivors.

VOLUME TWO

Dr Alyse Price-Tobler PhD

NATIONAL
LIBRARY
OF AUSTRALIA

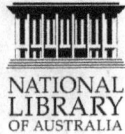

A catalogue record for this book is available from the National Library of Australia

A catalogue record for this book etc…

This book is non-fiction.

Book # : 2

Publisher:
Inspiring Publishers
P.O. Box 159, Calwell, ACT Australia 2905
Email: inspiringpublisher.com
http://www.inspiringpublishers.com

National Library of Australia Cataloguing-in-Publication entry

Author: Dr Alyse Price-Tobler PhD

Title: **Navigating the Maze During Treatment of Adult Survivors of Child Psychological Abuse: Severe Parental Alienation - Volume Two**
A Comprehensive Resource Guide for Mental Health Practitioners, Offering Insights, Strategies and Risk Mitigation from a PhD Thesis on the Challenges Faced by Practitioners Treating Adult Child Survivors.

ISBN: 978-1-923250-07-9 (print)
ISBN: 978-1-923250-08-6 (ePub2)

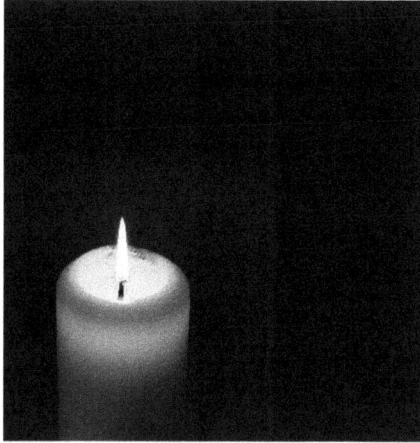

For my grandson Lyran James Tao Price

You are brave, you are strong, and you can be
anything you want to be in this lifetime

In times of confusion about the multiverse, draw upon
Mahatma Gandhi - "Be the change you wish to see in the world,"
and ALWAYS look for the light. Love Ma Mare xox

Acknowledgements

I want to take this opportunity to express my heartfelt gratitude to all the individuals who have supported me throughout my journey at The Sunshine Coast University.

First and foremost, I am especially indebted to my primary PhD supervisor, Dr Dyann Ross, and my secondary supervisor, Dr Peter Innes, for believing in my abilities to complete a PhD. Furthermore, I am incredibly grateful for the patience they have shown me as a mature student from a challenging educational background.

Special thanks go to my surrogate mother and wise counsellor, Patricia deLaney-Davis, who has been a maternal figure in my life for the past 30 years. She has provided unwavering support, guiding me through my challenges with compassion and selflessness. As a Catholic, Brigadine Sister, Trishy dedicated herself to serving the most vulnerable in society, embodying motherly compassion and selflessness as she worked tirelessly as a teacher and counsellor on the streets of Sydney to care for the homeless and those with mental health challenges for more than 30 years. Brigadine Sisters work in a variety of formal and informal ways as advocates for people who are marginalised in our world today – asylum seekers, refugees, travellers, indigenous and islander peoples and people vulnerable to being trafficked and exploited.

Trishy's unconditional love, which was always reminiscent of Mother Teresa to me, was a gift I had not experienced before meeting her and has been instrumental in my healing and professional journey in mental health and disabilities. With her guidance, I have integrated frontline skills, lived experiences, and academic qualifications, allowing me to make a meaningful difference in the lives of others. Her presence has been transformative, empowering me to achieve milestones such as obtaining my master's degree in 'primary homeless women experiencing severe and persistent mental health challenges' on Sydney streets, my doctorate in child psychological abuse and helping others navigate their own paths to healing in my private practice.

Thank you also to the universe and my family members who have passed for guiding me and keeping me safe. In particular, Dame Enid Lyons, whose father is my great-grandfather, from whom I have drawn inspiration throughout this journey. I pay homage to her and her words of wisdom when I think about the vulnerable people that I work with every day; "The problems of government were not problems of blue books, not problems of statistics, but problems of human values and human hearts and human feelings" (Henderson, 2018, p. xiii).

Thank you to my birth mother, Helen, for bringing me onto the earth to offer me the opportunity to try and heal our family's intergenerational trauma through my professional career and my thesis. The versions of love and pain you have shown me are now being reframed and adapted to help others.

My heartfelt appreciation goes to my darling husband, Shane, for all the time, unwavering practical support, cups of tea and love he has given me since I told him I was beginning a PhD. Thank you to my sister Kylie, my soul sister Dawn McCarty and my brother James for their staunch support and encouragement throughout this fascinating learning journey.

I also want to acknowledge my two beautiful, brave, strong children, Tristan and Alezandia, for their belief in my abilities and unconditional love. They have been my pillars of strength and provided me solace during challenging times. Thank you also to my beautiful, younger generation: Lily, Elizabeth, Rose, Isla, and especially my grandson Lyran, who was my inspiration and driving force to begin this journey.

Additionally, I extend my heartfelt gratitude to Dr. Craig Childress, a renowned clinical psychologist who has served as my clinical supervisor (for my private practice) over the past three years. His unwavering support and guidance in navigating my patients' challenges have been invaluable. Dr. Childress's expertise and mentorship have significantly enriched my professional development and clinical registration requirements. I sincerely appreciate his dedication, generosity, kindness, and encouragement throughout my journey, especially in helping me stay focused and balance my academic studies and work commitments separately.

Lastly, I would like to express my gratitude to all the adult survivors of 'severe level' child psychological abuse and the mental health practitioners who willingly volunteered their time, valuable perspectives, and expertise to contribute to my research. Their beneficial insights and willingness to share their experiences have significantly enriched the outcomes of these studies. Thank you for being integral to this incredible chapter in my life.

Dedication

I dedicate this thesis to three extraordinary men who died over eight weeks while writing this thesis between March and June 2021. The first was my beloved mentor of 30 years, Noel Davis (1943-2021), who embodied a profound sense of compassion and selflessness that left an indelible mark on my heart. Throughout his life, he tirelessly dedicated himself to serving the most vulnerable, offering solace and support to those who often went unnoticed and were in desperate need. Like a beacon of light in the darkness, Noel's gentle poetry, presence and unwavering kindness provided comfort and hope to the forlorn and lost. I was one of 'the lost' when I met Noel, and he saved my life twice. As a quiet and humble Marist brother, he lived out the teachings of Jesus, extending love and care to all he encountered, regardless of their circumstances. The values of the Marist Brothers are Presence, Simplicity, Family Spirit, Love of Work and following in The Way of Mary. Noels' legacy of compassion inspires me daily, reminding me of the power of kindness and the profound impact one individual can have on the world.

Secondly, my beloved father, Geoffrey Charles Bonner (1944-2021), was a man of quiet strength and unwavering love. Despite the challenges he faced, including the heartbreaking reality of being separated from me for 21 years due to parental alienation, he remained steadfast in his love and devotion. His intimate knowledge and lived experience of family and domestic violence aimed at him only served to deepen his compassion and empathy for others. Despite the pain he endured, my father's love knew no bounds. His passing, marked by 'unnatural causes,' left an ache in my heart that will never fully heal. Every day, I yearn for the lost years we could have shared, wishing for just a moment more to express the depth of my love. Though he may no longer be with me in body, his spirit lives on in the cherished memories we shared, and his enduring, unconditional love continues to inspire me with the work I do with my patients, now and always.

Lastly, my beloved uncle, Denis James Bonner (1946-2021), was foremost a conservatorium-trained pianist whose musical talent brought joy to all who heard him play. Despite grappling with severe and persistent mental health challenges, he found fulfilment in sharing his musical gift with the world. Later in life, Denis transitioned to a taxi driver and, with great pride, served as a Justice of the Peace. In his roles, he continued to touch lives, offering support and kindness to those who crossed his path in the inner city of Sydney. He became a mobile accidental counsellor, providing comfort and compassion to fellow outliers who found themselves in his taxi.

As I have had to bid farewell to these beloved figures in my life, I am reminded of the importance of breaking the cycle of intergenerational trauma that has plagued our family. I am committed to tirelessly fighting to end these destructive patterns for the sake of future generations. May my father Geoffrey, Uncle Denis, my paternal grandparents, Linda (Lindy Lou) and Charles, whom we were not allowed to see and my Uncle Peter (who died by suicide), all rest in peace, knowing that their legacy of love for us lives on in my twin academic thesis, psychological literature and educational material on severe level parental alienation/ child abuse.

With love and gratitude, Dr Alyse Price-Tobler, PhD, University of the Sunshine Coast.

Foreword

It is with great pleasure that I welcome another masterful work of research and clinical scholarship in a much-needed domain: the treatment of adult survivors of child psychological abuse by a pathological parent. Dr. Price-Tobler brings a wealth of professional and experiential knowledge as a clinical psychotherapist working on the front line of mental health treatment and disabilities for the past 38 years. Her prior Master's level clinical research focus was on women experiencing both homelessness and mental illness issues. Dr. Price-Tobler is passionate about going to our most vulnerable, identifying and treating the needs of those we abandon.

For her doctoral dissertation, Dr. Price-Tobler focused on another forgotten and neglected population, the now-adult survivors of child psychological abuse by a parent surrounding divorce and family conflict, often called "parental alienation" by the general public (DSM-5 300.19 Factitious Disorder Imposed on Another; 297.1 Delusional Disorder (shared), V995.51 Child Psychological Abuse). Through her doctoral studies, Dr Price-Tobler obtained twin PhD doctorates by her focus on both the child psychological abuse related to adult survivors of severe level "parental alienation" and the current approaches of the mental health practitioners who treat them therapeutically. This is the second instalment of her doctoral thesis that was entitled "Working with Adult-Child Survivors of Severe Parental Alienation Abuse: Survivors and Mental Health Practitioners Perspectives." In her second book, Dr. Price-Tobler provides her research-generated insights on the issues and struggles surrounding mental health practitioners and their treatment of now-adult survivors of fractured families and childhood psychological abuse by a parent.

Over the years, it has been my great pleasure to know and work with Dr. Price-Tobler as she followed her professional path into the family courts and the treatment of the child abuse that is there and that remains embedded in the now-adult survivors long after the custody battles of childhood are gone. Being an adult survivor of severe "parental alienation" as a child, including parental abduction, ultimately led her to embark on her twin study PhD to develop both a treatment protocol for the now-adult survivors, along with an examination of the mental health professionals who treat them and their needs. Through her own recovery from her childhood traumas, Dr. Price-Tobler found her voice in professional scholarship and in her passion for recovering the victims of child abuse who were not recovered during childhood – a forgotten population of child abuse victims from the family courts within a severely fractured family.

Working in the family courts is difficult, with many barriers and challenges, not only from the pathology in the family courts but also often from the professionals (for various reasons). Despite all the obstacles she has faced, Dr. Price-Tobler has been sustained by her passion for protecting children – of any age – from the ravages of child abuse. We never abandon a single child to child abuse, not even the now-adult ones.

Dr. Price-Tobler stands as a testament to recovery and more. Her professional accomplishments in clinical research and in bringing the light of knowledge to the darkness of children abandoned to child abuse are evidence not merely of her survival but of her victory over the traumas that tried to shape her destiny and failed. Her victory of emerging into professional leadership in the recovery of children (of any age) from childhood abuse should inspire all now-adult survivors of child abuse to reclaim their voices, their identities, and their unique "wild and precious lives" (Mary Oliver) from the abuse that tried to shape them – and failed.

The pathology in the family courts is tearing families apart and savaging the bonds of love within families, destroying not only childhoods but also the future lives of the children as adults. Dr. Price-Tobler works on the front lines of battle to protect children and recover healthy bonds of affection, love, and support throughout the family. The focus of the family courts is on the children in the family courts, but who helps the survivors of child abuse who were not protected, who were lost within the 'system'? The needs of the children in the family courts are substantial, as are the needs of the now-adult survivors who were not protected at the time and who now suffer the consequences in adulthood that result from untreated psychological abuse in childhood.

The psychological abuse of children by a pathological parent surrounding child custody conflict can leave lifelong scars to identity and future relationships. Yet even more severely devastating to development is when the pathology extends into child abduction surrounding divorce and custody conflict. The overlay of damage to the child from both pathological parenting and the terrors of abduction creates a particularly destructive variant of child abuse. As a personal survivor of childhood abduction, in addition to the surrounding psychological abuse by a pathological parent, Dr. Price-Tobler brings particular expertise and insights into understanding and treating a devasting form of child abuse.

The passions, experience, and professional scholarship of Dr. Price-Tobler now yield the second book from her dissertation regarding the work of mental health practitioners who provide treatment support for the adult survivors of child psychological abuse and the complex professional challenges associated with this work. In this, her second book, "Navigating the Maze During Treatment of Adult Survivors of Child Psychological Abuse: Severe Parental Alienation. A Comprehensive Resource Guide for Mental Health Practitioners, Offering Insights, Strategies, and Risk Mitigation from a PhD Thesis on the Challenges Faced by Practitioners Treating Adult Child Survivors. Volume Two," Dr. Alyse Price-Tobler sheds valuable light on the professional challenges, delving into the nuanced and often isolating experiences of these dedicated professionals. This book is not merely an academic exploration; it is an urgent call to action.

Dr. Price-Tobler's insight into the field of mental health treatment for psychological child abuse by a severely pathological parent stems originally from her own experiences with mental health professionals, and this childhood experience now informs her understanding of the role of mental health professionals in treatment and recovery. Throughout her formative years, Dr. Price-Tobler received the standard mental health involvement from many clinical psychologists. Yet, none of them could identify the psychological abuse she endured as a child. None of them could understand the complex family dynamics of severe "parental alienation" and abduction. Instead of recognising her abuse and trauma, these professionals aligned (and colluded) with her pathological mother against her father, misdiagnosing the child abuse and wrongly attributing the child's symptoms to the child cause rather than to the psychological child abuse she suffered from a pathological parent.

The personal history of Dr. Price-Tobler fuels her commitment to addressing the gaps in understanding and treatment within the mental health field. Her second book details the urgent need for clinically tested treatment protocols and specialised training to equip mental health practitioners, their clinical supervisors, and medical professionals with the knowledge and skills to effectively address the myriad of mental and physical health issues their clients face. The book explores the qualifications and specialty areas of specialist mental health practitioners who currently work with adult child survivors of child psychological abuse surrounding severe "parental alienation", delving into their backgrounds and demographics. Finally, she highlights the unique challenges faced by therapists with lived experience (TLE), the broader social impact of severe "parental alienation", the scope of complex intersecting traumas (CITs) reported by mental health practitioners, and the dire consequences that result from misdiagnosis and ineffective treatment, such as familicide, homicide, abduction, and parental threats of harm to the child.

Trauma treatment can be emotionally and psychologically stressful for the involved mental health professionals from both vicarious trauma and the isolation experienced by practitioners. Developing an appropriate professional support community will be important to treating the trauma pathology in the child and family by spreading the family's traumas across multiple system points through consultation and support. In her second book, Dr. Price-Tobler describes the physical, psychological, and mental health impacts on the professionals working with a particular form of psychological child abuse found in the family courts. Through her exceptional scholarship, Dr. Price-Tobler begins the process of identifying effective therapies and treatment modalities within the context of the professional and ethical challenges involved with treating court-involved child and family pathology.

Craig Childress, Psy.D.
Clinical Psychologist, CA PSY 18857

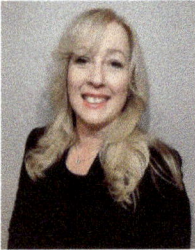

About the Author

Dr Alyse Price-Tobler, PhD, is an experienced mental health practitioner, academic researcher, and clinical psychotherapist (MCAP). She has recently completed her pioneering doctoral research on adult-child survivors who have suffered psychological abuse, also known as severe parental alienation, during their developmental years. Her study also focused on the mental health practitioners who support this group and their current treatment approaches. With a keen focus on severe parental alienation and abduction (SPAA), her work aims to understand and address the challenges faced by survivors while developing effective treatment protocols in this area. With 38 years of frontline experience in mental health and disabilities work, Dr Price-Tobler's journey is deeply personal, as she is an adult survivor of severe level parental alienation and abduction.

Masters Degree Research

Dr Price-Tobler's expertise extends to her active practice as a master's degree holder in psychotherapy and counselling (MCAP), where she researched women who were experiencing primary homelessness on the streets of Sydney while living with severe and persistent mental illness. Dr Price-Tobler works with diverse clients in her private practice, including NDIS and CALD clients and patients in mental health units.

Also, as a result of the data collected from her master's degree research with homeless women, Dr Price-Tobler designed the Sempi Social Communication Model (SSCM) as an answer to the question RUOK? The SSCM is a model designed to teach the general public how to be first responders to their community if someone is not OK and cannot access professional mental health help quickly. The SSCM is a free, altruistic, pay-it-forward model for children and adults at the grassroots level of communities worldwide. The 'SEMPI© Model' is written for everyone, regardless of disability, mental health challenge, occupation, or religion.

PhD Research

Her deep-seated dedication to understanding the intricacies of child psychological abuse stems from her own firsthand experiences. Central to her research is her twin PhD thesis titled "Working with Adult-Child Survivors of Severe Parental Alienation Abuse: Survivors and Mental Health Practitioners Perspectives," which delves into the complex challenges regarding current treatments within this field. Dr. Price-Tobler conducted thorough studies involving interviews with adult-child survivors of severe psychological abuse and ten of the world's foremost expert mental health practitioners specialising in severe parental alienation and abduction. These efforts have culminated in developing an innovative, soon-to-be-published treatment protocol.

Specialty Areas

Dr. Price-Tobler specialises in supporting a diverse range of individuals facing complex challenges. This includes adult child survivors and targeted parents experiencing severe levels of parental alienation, individuals dealing with complex disabilities, sex workers, internet addiction, family and domestic violence, juvenile justice offenders, including young offenders with disabilities charged with sexual offences, and those exhibiting sexualised behaviours to prevent such offences.

Additionally, she has expertise in addressing specific mental health concerns such as premenstrual dysphoric disorder (PMDD), coping with stillbirth, death, and dying, as well as managing suicidal ideation and suicide prevention. She also specialises in psychotherapy for severe mental health conditions such as schizophrenia, psychosis, familicide, and dissociative identity disorder (DID). Dr. Price-Tobler also leads a support group tailored for family members who have survived familicide events involving family members experiencing psychosis and schizophrenia. Furthermore, she extends her support to foster care and trafficked youth and primary homeless individuals, focusing on those who are disenfranchised and vulnerable.

Additionally, Dr Price-Tobler works with female offenders who have committed serious crimes against society before and after they are paroled, providing support and assistance in their rehabilitation process. She also educates male offenders on non-violent communication (Rosenberg, 2015) and appropriate interactions with women before their release, aiming to promote respectful and healthy relationships. Interestingly, many of these challenged community members are also adult child survivors of SPA. Lastly, these specialty focus areas are not just professional interests but represent the core of her work.

Professional Membership

Dr Price-Tobler is also a clinical member of PACFA Australia, the American Psychological Association, the Parental Alienation Study Group (PASG) and a founding member of the Australian-based Transcending Alienation Practitioners and Professionals Group (TAPP).

Volunteer work

University

In December 2023, the University of the Sunshine Coast awarded Dr Price-Tobler its 'Community Volunteer of the Year Award' for her mentorship and contributions to fellow PhD students. She also won a 'Student Leadership Award for 2023' for supporting other students in the Masters and higher degree by research PhD program at UniSC.

State Emergency Service

Furthermore, Dr Price-Tobler has dedicated 20 years to volunteer service in the NSW State Emergency Service (SES). During this time, she has fulfilled various first responder positions, such as serving as an active rescue officer and trainer. She has been involved in and facilitated numerous search and rescue missions involving heights, depths, caves, helicopters, large animals and primary road crashes. Additionally, she holds the highest rescue certification attainable in Australia.

Dr. Price-Tobler has been acknowledged for her bravery in several community disasters. However, the one she is proudest of was receiving recognition from the NSW Governor General for her efforts during the tragic Thredbo landslide, which claimed the lives of 18 people. With her extensive experience as a first responder and training officer with the NSW SES, Dr Price-Tobler also specialises in providing first responder crisis counselling, aiding volunteers in maintaining optimal mental and physical health during critical incidents and disasters as required.

Anti-Alienation Project

Dr Price-Tobler is also part of the advisory panel for the Anti-Alienation Project and voluntarily co-facilitates the adult survivors group, a project aimed at supporting and raising the voices of adult child survivors of child psychological abuse in the form of parental alienation. https://www.youtube.com/channel/UCfzOR3LLqL0fMtz_J_o4vjw

Humanly Possible Channel

Additionally, she co-founded and co-hosted the 'Facebook Humanly Possible Channel' with Dawn McCarty, a cyber security expert and fellow adult survivor of SPAA. Together, they leverage this platform to raise parental alienation awareness and share their experiences to foster understanding. https://www.facebook.com/HumanlyPossibleChannel

Contact

To connect with Dr Alyse Price-Tobler-

Email: drapricetobler@sempi.com.au
LinkedIn: (https://www.linkedin.com/in/alyse-price-tobler-135459114/)
Twitter: (https://twitter.com/AlyseTobler)
Youtube: https://www.youtube.com/channel/
               UCiN_DxTEdbOpGZNB3Bo3ndQ/videos
Website: For more information on individual trauma counselling and onsite counselling retreat packages, go to www.alyseprice-tobler.com
The SEMPI Social Communication Model - https://www.sempi.net

Abstract

The issue of childhood exposure to severe levels of child psychological abuse related to parental alienation is a prevalent and serious problem that can have long-lasting adverse effects on adult survivors. This research has addressed this issue, highlighting its significance in understanding the challenges faced by survivors and the specialist mental health practitioners (MHPs) who support them. However, MHPs are often ill-equipped to work with survivors due to limited training, professional development, and the lack of an established best-practice treatment protocol.

In response to this gap, the Researcher has developed a proposed treatment framework/theoretical treatment model, which will be published in Volume Three. This framework draws from their expertise in studying the adult child survivor cohort, the mental health practitioner cohort, and the integration of their lived experience and is informed by their work as a mental health practitioner who has professionally served on the frontline in the field of disabilities and mental health for 38 years.

In Volume One, the associated research delves into the perspectives of adult-child survivors of psychological abuse associated with severe parental alienation (SPA) regarding their treatment by MHPs. Volume Two will present data from the thesis, focusing on the current perspectives and treatments being applied by the world-leading international MHPs specialising in trauma therapy for these survivors. These perspectives inform both effective and ineffective mental health practices while exploring the hurdles encountered by MHPs when working with survivors. This comprehensive approach provides a deeper understanding of the multifaceted dynamics within therapeutic and related environments.

Note: The term 'adult-child survivor' denotes an individual exposed to child psychological abuse related to SPA during their formative years. Parental alienation (PA) encompasses the deliberate actions of an alienating parent (AP) negatively impacting the child's relationship with their targeted parent (TP). In instances of SPA, where child survivors endure heightened psychological abuse, symptoms may have escalated to distressing levels. For instance, children who are experiencing SPA exhibit adamant hostility, refuse visits and even express threats to run away. An unhealthy alliance forms with the AP, leading to the destruction of the parent-child relationship and the manifestation of intense hostility, including paranoid delusions and unfounded apprehensions of potential harm or violence (Baker, 2007).

In light of the ongoing historical turmoil, Study Two adopted a research methodology rooted in a social constructionist thematic analysis approach and a qualitative research design. This volume presents findings from semi-structured interviews conducted as part of the associated twin PhD thesis. For example, the ten MHP participants collectively held fifty-seven qualifications, spanning multiple specialty areas or professions. Most practitioners reported over fifteen years of experience in mental health, with several years of advanced-level practice. The combined professional experience of the study participants in the mental health sector totalled two hundred and sixty-seven years.

The findings of Study Two highlight the ambiguity of MHPs' experiences regarding the appropriate course of treatment and reveal that MHPs utilise a combination of therapeutic approaches. In the data collection process, ten MHPs reported implementing thirty-seven preferred therapeutic modalities and therapies when working with survivors. Thus, the data suggests a considerable degree of diversity in the therapeutic approaches used to address the needs of survivors among the practitioners. This diversity in approaches raises essential questions about the efficacy of existing treatment practices.

Furthermore, the MHPs reported experiencing vicarious trauma, which they believed manifested as physical and mental health issues. This trauma stemmed from listening to the survivors' traumatic accounts and enduring experiences resulting from working within the Family Court system, the actions of PA opponents, other parental alienation professionals, TPs and APs.

In addition to the trauma experienced by MHPs regarding survivors' traumatic accounts and enduring the consequences of actions by various individuals involved in PA, an intriguing finding emerged regarding the interaction between clinical supervisors and MHP supervisees. The research reveals that supervisees receiving clinical supervision regarding SPA clients are paradoxically teaching clinical supervisors about PA and SPA.

Also, even when they teach their clinical supervisors about SPA, the supervisors become 'burnt out' and choose not to work with the MHP anymore, consequently leaving specialist SPA MHPs without clinical supervision and at risk of psychological harm to themselves. Other MHPs discussed the threat of deregistration if they did not meet their required clinical supervision hours.

This finding is particularly noteworthy because it illustrates a concerning pattern. It demonstrates that when supervisees, especially those working with survivors of SPA, participate in mandated clinical supervision sessions to uphold their registration, clinical supervisors can experience burnout. This can result in supervisees being unable to gain the necessary supervision to maintain their accreditation and may lead some to resort to dishonest practices, such as falsifying supervision requirements to keep working with SPA clients or potentially, they may burn themselves out.

Additionally, the connection between clinical supervisors discontinuing the supervision of MHPs and the potential departure of MHPs from their clients who are adult survivors is evident for several reasons. Interestingly, adult survivors participating in the research expressed a crucial need to educate their therapists about child psychological abuse and the specific dynamics of complex intersecting traumas (CITs) they have encountered so they could get the help that they required. The adult survivors expressed that failure to address these needs in session may lead therapists to disengage from working with survivors, leaving them without the necessary support. This underscores a shared vulnerability between clinical supervisors and MHPs, both of whom face the risk of leaving their roles due to the challenges associated with working with survivors of SPA.

Besides the lack of clinical supervision, MHPs might also stop seeing survivors due to feeling overwhelmed or unsupported in managing the complexities of the survivors' experiences. Additionally, personal or professional challenges, such as experiencing vicarious trauma or facing organisational constraints, can affect their ability to provide continued support to survivors.

These results suggest a broader issue of disharmony within the field, underlining the necessity for further dialogue and standardisation in SPA training and practice. For instance, among the MHP participants, 72 suggestions for 'other' treatments were provided, shedding light on the current practices employed by MHPs when working with adult survivors of SPA. Interestingly, only five subjects were repeated among the seventy-two subjects examined, while the remaining sixty-seven recommended subjects were mentioned only once.

This finding is particularly intriguing given that seven MHPs had experience working with survivors from mild to severe levels and three specialised in severe cases. However, despite their varying levels of experience, most of them lacked specific formal training in the intricate dynamics of child psychological abuse, also referred to as pathogenic parenting, associated with attachment-based parental alienation (Childress, 2015).

Moreover, an interesting observation emerged among the MHP study participants: Each recommended different subjects to their counterparts. This lack of overlap or repetition in the recommended subjects indicates an absence of consensus among the participants, suggesting that no universally agreed-upon set of subjects considered relevant for MHPs in the SPA profession exists.

Furthermore, the wide range of recommended subjects underscores the diverse perspectives among SPA MHPs, with each participant likely drawing from their own experiences, prior knowledge, or personal beliefs. This diversity reflects the multifaceted nature of CITs in SPA and the various approaches and knowledge bases MHPs bring to the field. Samples of these findings will be discussed in Volume Two. However, the complete findings will be detailed, applied, and expanded upon in Volume Three, featuring the proposed treatment framework for mental health practitioners to use when assisting adult child survivors.

On a different note, it is worth stating that in Study Two, an intriguing discovery was uncovered where 50% of the MHPs participating in the research identified themselves as highly qualified lived experience therapists who had personally experienced trauma. Moreover, these professionals intend to inform their clients about their lived experiences if they deem it relevant. This discovery contradicts prevalent training resources, which frequently advise MHPs against disclosing personal details to clients to maintain professionalism when the MHP considers it necessary. It also challenges other literature that emphasises the stigma faced by MHPs who openly acknowledge their own personal experiences.

Furthermore, it is essential for MHPs to be aware that the Researcher of these studies also noted two potentially new clinical findings while coding the adult survivor data. Specifically, three of the four survivor participants (75%) who had undergone 'SPA and abduction' (SPAA) during their early childhood (under eight years old) described an unusual 'specific phobia, anxiety variant' that was not previously researched or reported in the existing child or adult SPA literature according to the Researcher's knowledge.

Consequently, this finding may carry clinical significance, given the limited research on the effects of 'SPA' and 'abduction' on children under eight. It is worth noting that specific phobias related to 'SPA' and 'abduction' are usually researched separately and are scarcely mentioned in the literature. Furthermore, there is a dearth of information when these terms are directly connected. Therefore, the Researcher has named the new variant 'specific phobia-severe parental alienation, and abduction anxiety variant' (Price-Tobler, 2023).

It is imperative to highlight these findings to MHPs so that further research can be conducted, and they can be vigilant in identifying and treating the 'specific phobia-severe parental alienation and abduction anxiety variant'. By bringing attention to this potentially unreported clinical phenomenon, MHPs can contribute to expanding their understanding of the effects of SPAA on children under eight, ultimately enhancing their ability to provide comprehensive and effective treatment for survivors. Please refer to Volume One for more details.

Secondly, the 'specific phobia-severe parental alienation and abduction anxiety variant' may represent a direct link between severe parental alienation and factitious disorder imposed on another (FDIOA), previously described as Munchausen by proxy and also potentially shared delusional disorder (SDD). The Researcher suggests that survivors of SPAA in these studies may have been exposed to a parent who actively engaged in FDIOA or shared delusional disorder, involving the deliberate exaggeration or fabrication of a child's psychological or physical condition with the intention to deceive (American Psychiatric Association, 2013). While FDIOA is commonly associated with physical presentations, it is crucial to acknowledge that some APs can also inflict psychological harm on their children. This potential connection highlights the complexity and severity of psychological abuse within

SPAA cases and underscores the importance of further research and awareness among MHPs.

The results from these studies underscore the urgent need for further research and enhanced professional development opportunities in the domain of SPA. They also emphasise the critical role of equipping MHPs with the necessary tools and expertise to support adult survivors effectively. The Researcher will leverage these studies to develop protocols for MHPs who treat survivors, ultimately improving mental health outcomes and enhancing the long-term well-being of this population.

While the current research offers valuable insights into the experiences of adult-child survivors of SPA and SPAA and the challenges encountered by MHPs, it is essential to acknowledge certain limitations. Due to the data indicating potential links and exposure of SPAA survivors to FDIOA and SDD, this unexpected finding underscores the complex and multifaceted nature of PA and the diverse forms of trauma that adult-child survivors may have endured. However, it is important to note that the exploration of FDIOA and SDD falls outside the predefined scope of this research.

These studies advocate recognising and addressing the unique needs of MHPs, emphasising the psychological impact of working in this field. The studies underscore the imperative for further research and professional development in SPA and SPAA across various areas, aiming to equip MHPs with the knowledge and tools necessary to support adult-child survivors effectively. Additionally, the present findings lay the groundwork for clinical trials to develop an evidence-based treatment protocol tailored for adult-child survivors, which may be better than the protocol suggested by the Researcher in Volume Three.

Lastly, within the anomalous data, the Researcher discovered that, concerningly, one MHP study participant reported that five MH professionals at their place of work have cancer, which they believe relates to working in the PA field, and another one (equalling six) was experiencing aggressive leukaemia. Important note: In discussing the previously described data in these studies, it is important to acknowledge certain caveats. Firstly, the Researcher reports that the data presented represents the MHPs' perspectives on cancer among their peers. It is crucial to recognise that data from these studies may not have reached the level of support typically expected in rigorous research. However, it serves as a valuable starting point for future investigations to build upon.

Note from the author: Despite my professional collaboration with Dr. Childress for clinical supervision and mentoring over the past three years, I acknowledge the potential for perceived bias. However, drawing from my personal experiences as an adult child who endured severe parental alienation and abduction, coupled with my background as a researcher and professional mental health practitioner, my commitment lies in presenting all facts objectively and seeking accurate diagnoses and treatments for adult children affected by SPA and abduction.

Furthermore, in the face of challenging circumstances, the Researcher has made a difficult decision. Rather than pursuing funding and the lengthy process of designing clinical trials, they have prioritised publishing their treatment framework in Volume Three. This decision reflects an acknowledgment of the urgency of recognising that individuals affected by SPA and SPAA cannot afford to wait for potentially life-saving interventions. As a single individual, the Researcher is determined to make a meaningful difference in the lives of those impacted by this complex phenomenon.

Table of Contents

✦

List of Figures

List of Tables

Table 1	Extract from Adult Survivor and MHP Interview Transcripts	Refer to Volume One
Table 2	Adult Survivor Participant Demographics	Refer to Volume One
Table 3	Therapies Applied by MHPs to Adult Survivors as Stated by Survivors	Refer to Volume One
Table 4	Ideas, Topics, and Psychoeducation as Recommended by Survivors	Refer to Volume One
Table 5	Mental and Physical Health Challenges Reported by MHPs	Page 104-108

List of Appendices

Disrupting the Intergenerational Trauma Cycle

Abbreviations and Acronyms

Acronyms	
ABPA	Attachment-Based Parental Alienation
ACES	Adverse Childhood Experiences
ACE's	Adverse Childhood Experiences Study
BSQ	Baker Strategy Questionnaire
CITs	Complex Intersecting Traumas
CSA	Child Sexual Abuse
CTT	Contemporary Trauma Theory
FDIOA	Factitious Disorder Imposed On Another
FDV	Family and Domestic Violence
IPV	Intimate Partner Violence
MH	Mental Health
MHP	Mental Health Practitioner
MHPs	Mental Health Practitioners
MRSA	Methicillin-resistant Staphylococcus aureus
PA	Parental Alienation
PABs	Parental Alienating Behaviours
PAS	Parental Alienation Syndrome

SPA	Severe Parental Alienation
SPAA	Severe Parental Alienation and Abduction
SDD	Shared Delusional Disorder
TIC	Trauma Informed Care

Please note that abbreviations and acronyms that were only mentioned once or twice were not included in this table.

Statement of Original Authorship

This thesis *is composed of my original work and contains* no material previously published or written by another person except where due reference has been made in the text. I have not engaged an editor to help me with this thesis.

I have clearly stated the contribution of others to my thesis as a whole, including statistical assistance, survey design, data analysis, significant technical procedures, professional editorial advice, financial support and any other original research work used or reported in my thesis. The content of my thesis is the result of work I have carried out since the commencement of my higher degree by research candidature and does not include a substantial part of work that has been submitted *to qualify for the award of any* other degree or diploma in any university or other tertiary institution. I have clearly stated which parts of my thesis, if any, have been submitted to qualify for another award.

I acknowledge that an electronic copy of my thesis must be lodged with the University Library and, subject to the policy and procedures of The University of the Sunshine Coast, the thesis be made available for research and study in accordance with the Copyright Act 1968 unless a period of embargo has been approved by the Dean of Graduate Research.

I acknowledge that the copyright of all material contained in my thesis resides with the copyright holder(s) of that material. Where appropriate, I have obtained copyright permission from the copyright holder to reproduce material in this thesis and have sought permission from co-authors for any jointly authored works included in the thesis.

Finally, this thesis was solely prepared and edited by the author. No professional editors or external assistants were involved in this work's writing, editing, or content development.

Alyse Price-Tobler *18.8.23*

Financial Support

I also acknowledge that this research was supported by an Australian Government Research Training Program Scholarship, which I deeply appreciate for its contribution to the realisation of this research endeavour.

Ethics Approval
for Research

Human research ethics approval for the research project: Working with Adult Survivors of Severe Parental Alienation: Survivors and Mental Health Practitioners Perspectives. A Qualitative Study (S211642).

Human subjects were involved in this research.

The Researcher applied for and was granted ethics approval with the University of the Sunshine Coast to follow appropriate scientific protocol. Ethical clearance was obtained from the National Health and Medical Research Council (NHMRC) through the Human Research Ethics Application (HREA), approval number S211642.

A letter of approval was sent on December 21, 2021, by A/Prof Andrew Crowden, Chair, Human Research Ethics Committee Tel: +61 7 5430 2823 Email: humanethics@usc.edu.au

The letter of approval is included in Appendix Ten.

Keywords

The keywords for this thesis were Parental Alienation, ACEs, Adult, Adult Children, Anxiety, Child Abuse, Conflict, Depression, Mental Health Practitioners, and Parental Conflict.

Welcome to Volume Two

Dear Adult Child Survivors and MHPs,

Welcome to Volume Two of our exploration into the intricate landscape of trauma and its psychological underpinnings. While primarily tailored for mental health practitioners seeking to deepen their understanding and refine their understanding of this phenomenon, this volume extends an invitation to another vital cohort: adult child survivors grappling with the aftermath of trauma.

Within these pages, we delve into the complexities of trauma's impact on the human psyche, offering insights and strategies informed by contemporary psychological research and clinical practice. While the content may sometimes appear specialised, its relevance extends beyond the confines of professional discourse. Adult child survivors, who bear the indelible marks of early trauma, may find within these chapters a source of validation, illumination, and empowerment. By delving into the psychological mechanisms underlying their experiences, survivors can better understand their reactions, behaviours, and emotional responses.

Furthermore, the insights gleaned from this exploration may guide the path toward healing and self-discovery. Empowered with knowledge, adult survivors can forge a more profound connection with their inner selves and navigate the complexities of their journey with greater resilience. Moreover, for adult child survivors, sharing these volumes with their mental health practitioners can catalyse a collaborative journey toward healing.

By equipping therapists with the insights contained herein, survivors can empower them to navigate the intricacies of child psychological abuse, fostering a more informed and effective therapeutic alliance. May Volume One and Two serve as beacons of hope, understanding, and transformation for all seeking to help survivors or recover from trauma's enduring shadow.

The Joy of Being Ourselves

A Poem By Noel Davis (1943-2021)

How wonderful it is to feel ourselves
coming home to ourselves
approving, delighting, loving ourselves
forgiving ourselves of our wrongdoing
learning the lessons of our failures.

In spending time with our inner youngster
delighting in our inner child
feeling forgiven and encouraging forgiveness
there flows the joy of life
and the joy of seeing in a fresh new way.

How good to be coming home
feeling loved and less afraid of what might come
forgiven for being a wild thing
and playing in our Sunday best.

As we jettison life's debris
life the anchor of the past
leave behind it's drag on us
let fade the trauma of our scars
we make space for the joy
of coming home to ourselves (Davis, 2022).

✧
Introduction

Volume One of the associated twin PhD study provided new insights into the experiences of now adult-child survivors who endured intense conflicts between their parents during their childhood. These individuals were subjected to severe psychological abuse by a pathological parent (Childress, 2015), a phenomenon termed severe parental alienation (SPA) in this research. This type of parent is commonly involved in family court systems and is recognised as one of the most dangerous pathologies on earth (Childress, 2015).

Parental alienation (PA) remains prevalent in both professional and public discourse. It describes the process whereby one parent, often identified as the pathological or alienating parent (AP), undermines the relationship between the child and the targeted parent (TP) (Haines et al., 2020, p. 3). This concept is defined as the APs' behaviours influencing the child to reject the TP without a reasonable explanation (Haines et al., 2020).

Additionally, in cases where survivors have experienced SPA, the psychological abuse toward them from the pathogenic parent (Childress, 2015) has been more extreme, forcing the survivor's symptoms to manifest to distressing levels and continue into adulthood. For example, children experiencing SPA abuse are adamant in their hatred towards the TP, refusing visits and even threatening to run away (Baker, 2007). They develop an unhealthy alliance with the AP, sharing paranoid fantasies about the TP, leading to the relationship's destruction (Baker, 2007). Some children experiencing SPA can exhibit extreme hostility, including paranoid delusions and baseless fears of being harmed or murdered (Gardner, 2008, p. 2).

However, it is important to note that these terms are contentious among PA experts. In light of the ongoing discourse among professional PA experts regarding terminology, the Researcher advises that readers of this book maintain an open-minded approach to ideas concerning the assessment and diagnosis of this intricate pathology. Given that we are still in the pioneering phase of treatment development and public understanding of this complex issue, it is crucial to prioritise emotional intelligence over succumbing to politics. By fostering collaboration and unity rather than division, we can collectively work towards resolving conflicts within the field, conquering PA and stopping the associated suicide within the adult survivor and targeted parent community.

Suggestions regarding new terminology, such as 'pathogenic parenting,' are briefly included to address this controversy and enhance clinical accuracy. Understanding the gravity of this pathology, Dr Craig Childress (2015) proposes a shift from the term 'parental alienation' to 'pathogenic parenting,' emphasising the profound impact of distorted parenting practices on the child's psychological well-being. Dr. Childress (2015) states that the term 'parental alienation' lacks a defined clinical construct. Instead, the more accurate clinical term is 'pathogenic parenting,' which describes parenting practices so aberrant and distorted that they produce significant psychopathology in the child. This term is primarily used in the context of distortions to the child's attachment system, as dysfunctional attachment arises in response to problematic parenting. Dr. Childress (2015) advises mental health professionals to transition toward using 'pathogenic parenting' to describe the pathology associated with an attachment-based model of parental alienation.

Dr Childress (2015) offers that as an alternative label for this complex pathology, mental health professionals may consider linking 'pathogenic parenting' and 'parental alienation' to specify the associated type of pathogenic parenting, resulting in the combined phrase 'pathogenic parenting associated with attachment-based parental alienation' as a more accurate label to prevent the concealment of child abuse in family courts. Dr Childress (2024) emphasises that euphemisms for child abuse, such as 'parental alienation', 'resist refuse dynamics', and 'parent-child contact problems', are problematic. Professionals should acknowledge them as such to effectively treat this pathology (Childress, 2024). Furthermore, he also reports that diagnosis guides treatment, and euphemisms used in the family court system obscure the reality of child psychological abuse.

This discussion on euphemisms is vital in today's context. It provides 'grist for the mill', where there's a growing recognition of the importance of clear and accurate language, particularly in addressing sensitive issues like child psychological abuse. The Researcher purports that if the term 'parental alienation' is considered a euphemism, does it downplay the severity of emotional manipulation, coercion, and psychological abuse, obscuring the true harm inflicted upon the child and targeted parent? Additionally, does this euphemistic language undermine efforts to address the complex dynamics of abuse, perpetuating harm and hindering effective intervention, especially in the Family Court system?

Dr Childress notes specific diagnostic codes in the DSM-5 and ICD-10CM related to child psychological abuse and spouse or partner abuse, emphasising the importance of recognising these forms of abuse in clinical practice (Childress, 2024). These include:

Delusional Disorder-persecutory type (shared) DSM-5 297.1 - ICD - 10CM F22.

Factitious Disorder Imposed on Another DSM-5 300.19 - ICD 10 CM F68.10.

Child Psychological Abuse DSM - 5 V995.51 - ICD - 10 CM T74.32.

Spouse or Partner Abuse, Psychological DSM - 5 V995.82 - ICD - 10 CM Z69.11.

Interestingly, the prevalence of the term 'parental alienation' persists despite its challenges, largely because it strikes a chord with both the general public and adult survivors, fostering a preliminary understanding that can be deepened with further education. As individuals become more informed, they can promptly identify instances of PA, thus contributing to greater community awareness and understanding. Additionally, grasping the concept of PA opens the door to recognising it as a form of child psychological abuse, further enriching comprehension of the issue.

The term's widespread use within grassroots movements provides an avenue for additional education, bolstering understanding and advocacy efforts. By advocating for precise terminology, transparency, accountability, and better outcomes for those affected by child abuse can be promoted. However, it is important to note that despite its controversy, the term "parental alienation" is still commonly used, favoured by adult child survivors who are lay persons and others with degrees in psychology for its understanding of their trauma and its accessibility to the general public.

Moving forward, leveraging the term's widespread use within grassroots movements offers an opportunity for further education, strengthening understanding and advocacy endeavours. By championing precise terminology, we can foster transparency, accountability, and improved outcomes for individuals impacted by child psychological abuse.

Chapter Six
Results From the Twin PhD Thesis, Study Two: Mental Health Practitioners

Introduction

A social constructionist thematic analysis was employed in this exploratory research to investigate treatment modalities for MHPs working with survivors. The aim was to generate new data that can increase knowledge for MHPs who may work professionally with this population. A paucity of research on this subject prompted the decision to investigate the perspectives of MHPs who work with survivors. The findings of these studies contribute to the limited comparable data available for MHPs who specialise in working with children but lack sufficient information on treating adults who have experienced PA in all its forms, as reported in Volume One.

Volume Two presents an extensive exploration of topics relevant to the study of adult survivors of child psychological abuse, also known as severe parental alienation (SPA). The chapter delves into various facets of this complex issue, beginning with an examination of the areas of the brain affected by trauma and the neurochemicals impacted in infants. It then progresses to discuss the emotional manipulation techniques leading to brainwashing, drawing parallels between cult dynamics and SPA and elucidating the tactics used to brainwash adult survivors during their childhood.

Moreover, the chapter provides a detailed analysis of the specialty areas practised by mental health practitioners (MHPs), shedding light on their backgrounds, countries of origin, and genders. It also explores the role of therapists with lived experience (TLE) and family reunification practitioners alongside the motivations driving professionals to engage in the SPA field. Additionally, Volume Two investigates the number of SPA cases MHPs have encountered professionally and evaluates the broader societal impact of SPA.

Volume Two delves into key themes such as SPA and the associated Complex Intersecting Trauma (CIT) reported to MHPs, encompassing phenomena such as familicide, abduction, and threats of being killed. It also offers samples of the modalities and therapies practised by MHPs, offering insights into integrated treatment approaches and counselling methods while also considering ethical considerations inherent in this field.

Volume Two concludes with a sample series of recommendations for professional training and development, addressing gaps in knowledge, strategies to mitigate vicarious trauma, challenges encountered in the SPA field, and fostering collaborative dynamics among PA professionals. Volume Two also offers a thorough examination of severe levels of child psychological abuse and its manifestation in adult survivors, providing insights into the multifaceted dimensions of this issue. Additionally, it explores the impact on MHPs working with this population, shedding light on their challenges. Furthermore, the volume discusses the implications of severe child psychological abuse for mental health practice and research, highlighting the significant gaps in this field.

Qualifications of Mental Health Practitioners

Within Figure Eight, the combined number of MHPs' qualifications reported during the interview stage totalled fifty-seven. MHPs cited qualifications in more than one specialty area or profession. Most practitioners reported having over fifteen years of experience in mental health and added that they have been practising at an advanced level in their careers for several years. The combined years of the study participants' professional experience working in the mental health sector totalled two hundred and sixty-seven based on years reported during data collection. The combined qualifications of MHPs are presented in Figure Eight.

The Neurobiology of Trauma

The Researcher provides background information on the neurobiology of trauma experienced by adult survivors of child psychological abuse to contextualise the findings of the mental health practitioners (MHPs). The Researcher purports that understanding the neurobiological underpinnings of trauma is crucial for comprehending the long-term effects of child maltreatment. As De Bellis (2001, p. 539) suggests, child maltreatment can be considered an environmentally induced complex developmental disorder and may be a significant contributor to mental illness in both children and adults. Moreover, De Bellis (2001, p. 539) asserts that "child maltreatment may be the single most preventable and intervenable contributor to child and adult mental illness in this country."

Additionally, the epidemiology of maltreatment trauma is defined as repeated or sustained exposure to events that involve a betrayal of trust (De Bellis, 2001, as cited in Teicher & Samson, 2013, p. 1115). By exploring how trauma impacts areas of the brain associated with behaviour control, the neurochemical effects on infants, emotional manipulation leading to brainwashing, and the parallels between cult tactics and the severe parental alienation (SPA) strategies employed to manipulate adult survivors during childhood (Baker, 2007), the Researcher sets the stage for understanding the challenges faced by adult survivors. This understanding serves as a foundation for interpreting the results of the thesis on MHPs, who play a critical role in supporting these survivors.

This chapter examines how these findings intersect with the neurobiology of trauma experienced by adult survivors of child psychological abuse, shedding light on the complex developmental implications of maltreatment. Furthermore, it underscores the critical link between clinical interventions and biological mechanisms in understanding the impact of childhood trauma. Illustrating these dynamics, examples described as 'active' include childhood emotional, sexual, and physical abuse (Teicher & Samson, 2013). Conversely, examples described as 'passive' encompass physical and emotional neglect (Teicher & Samson, 2013).

The experience of trauma contributes to both short-term acute stress reactions and long-lasting neurobiological effects on the adult survivor (Cahill & Alkire, 2003). Alexander (2015) emphasises the importance for practitioners to comprehend the essence of maltreatment and break the cycle of violence. By learning how to maintain positive relationships while providing "an experience of emotional support," practitioners assist abuse survivors in developing resilience and protective factors (Alexander, 2015, pp. 8-9).

Research has underscored the impact of trauma on specific brain regions and neurochemicals, highlighting "enhanced human long-term memory consolidation produced with a naturally occurring stress hormone (epinephrine)" (Cahill & Alkire, 2003, p. 197). Furthermore, studies have shown that stressful events generating emotionally arousing experiences activate hormones within brain structures, facilitating the formation of strong memories (Bahtiyar et al., 2020). The synergistic action of glucocorticoid and norepinephrine hormones is believed to strengthen these memories, which are typically adaptive and vital for a child's survival (Bahtiyar et al., 2020). However, "aberrant memory processing of stressful events is a major risk factor for the development of stress-related psychopathology" and can result in maladaptive outcomes (Bahtiyar et al., 2020, p. 1). Strong fear memories are identified as significant risk factors for the development of fear-related disorders such as posttraumatic stress disorder (PTSD) and phobias (De Quervain et al., 2017, p. 7).

Areas of the Brain Affected by Trauma

Examining the role of fear memories in the development of such disorders provides insight into the broader impact of trauma on various brain regions. The human body relies on several systems to regulate specific behaviours. Among them are the limbic system, responsible for functions such as caregiving, dominance, cooperation, sexual mating, and care-seeking, and the reptilian brain, which supports bodily homeostasis (Alexander, 2015).

Furthermore, the neocortex is responsible for the creation of meaning (Alexander, 2015). Biologically, the limbic system and attachment are intertwined, ensuring that a child's proximity to their caregiver is vital for survival, particularly in times of danger (Alexander, 2015). When a child seeks attachment and their needs are met, proximity-seeking attachment behaviour diminishes, allowing the child to explore their surroundings (Alexander, 2015). The caregiver serves as both a secure base and a safe haven for the child during moments of fear or stress (Alexander, 2015).

From an evolutionary perspective, a child's attachment to a caregiver is inevitable for survival, given the necessity of the caregiver's attention and affection (Alexander, 2015). However, if a child experiences abandonment or neglect from their caregiver, it can instigate a realistic fear response, prompting the child to seek and maintain a constant connection with the caregiver, especially in perceived threatening situations (Alexander, 2015).

Attachment theory encompasses cognitive and affective aspects, highlighting the crucial role of a mother's ability to accurately perceive and respond to her child's emotional cues in shaping the development of the child's brain and identity (Alexander, 2015). Additionally, the process of mutual gaze and the mother's monitoring of her infant's facial expressions can synchronise their autonomic nervous systems, eliciting parallel sympathetic cardiac acceleration followed by parasympathetic cardiac deceleration in response to each other's smiles (Schore, 2002).

The primary site within the brain for synchronisation between the mother and infant is the right hemisphere of the brain, known as the orbitofrontal (ventromedial) cortex (Alexander, 2015). It is also known as "the thinking part of the emotional brain", functioning as the executive control centre for the whole right brain (Schore, 2002, p. 14). The right hemisphere is known for being in control of a "sense of physical and emotional self" and an "individual's awareness of his or her corporeal being and its relation to the environment and affective state" (Devinsky, 2000, p. 60). The right hemisphere also dominates our awareness pertaining to our physical and emotional self and the neural programs interpreting our body image in relation to our environment (Devinsky, 2000).

Additionally, a primary function of the right orbitofrontal cortex is to regulate the fear learning (Coan, 2008) response sent out from the amygdala by decreasing the sense of threat to the infant or expanding it (Alexander, 2015). The amygdala is very sensitive to facial cues, and when combined with the hippocampus, both positive and negative memories can be consolidated (Alexander, 2015). The hippocampus is an extension of the temporal part of the cerebral cortex. It is part of the limbic lobe (limbic means border), also known as the primitive brain, concerned with hunger, sex drive, motivation, pain, pleasure, mood, memory and appetite (Anand & Dhikav, 2012). It has a significant role in learning and memory and can be adversely affected by neurological and psychiatric disorders (Anand & Dhikav, 2012).

Scientific studies have highlighted the effects of childhood maltreatment and the relation that this abuse has to an increased risk of onset psychiatric disorders in adult survivors, such as substance abuse, major depression, anxiety disorders, and PTSD (Teicher & Samson, Childhood Maltreatment and Psychopathology: A Case for Ecophenotypic Variants as Clinically and Neurobiologically Distinct Subtypes, 2013). Furthermore, infants who have experienced child psychological abuse also referred to as parental alienation, may indeed be affected by the dynamics described. Parental alienation can disrupt the secure attachment bond between the child and the targeted parent, potentially leading to a sense of insecurity and fear in the child. If the alienating parent undermines the child's relationship with the targeted parent or creates a hostile environment, the child may experience emotional distress and may struggle to form healthy attachments. This can impact the child's ability to regulate emotions, form trusting relationships, and develop a secure sense of self.

Additionally, the absence of a secure attachment figure may hinder the child's ability to cope with stress and navigate social interactions effectively. Overall, parental alienation can have significant implications for the emotional and psychological well-being of infants and children. Moreover, these challenges can extend to the neurochemical level, impacting how infants respond to stress and perceive threats.

Neurochemicals Affected by Trauma in Infants

When an infant perceives a threat, the hypothalamus releases corticotropin-releasing hormone, triggering the release of adrenocorticotropic hormone into the pituitary gland. This process increases cortisol and catecholamine production in the adrenal cortex, prompting the infant's body to optimise function to cope with the perceived stress (Pier et al., 2016). The cortisol circulating in the infant's brain activates glucocorticoid receptors within the hippocampus, creating a feedback loop that inhibits hypothalamus-pituitary-adrenal axis (HPA) activity (Coan, 2008).

Over the past decade, compelling evidence has emerged regarding the critical role of glucocorticoids in memory consolidation, extinction, retrieval, and reconsolidation (De Quervain et al., 2017). These processes are highly relevant in developing and maintaining therapy for fear-related disorders stemming from child maltreatment (De Quervain et al., 2017).

From the research and analysis of journal articles, the Researcher suggests that adult survivors of parental alienation and child psychological abuse may experience persistent alterations in their stress response systems. These alterations can lead to heightened sensitivity to stress, difficulty regulating emotions, and dysregulation of the hypothalamus-pituitary-adrenal (HPA) axis.

Furthermore, chronic stress and trauma during childhood may impact brain regions involved in emotion regulation and memory processing, contributing to challenges in forming secure attachments and coping with stress in adulthood. The long-term consequences may include the development of fear-related disorders such as post-traumatic stress disorder (PTSD) and anxiety disorders. Overall, the findings underscore the profound and lasting impact of parental alienation and child psychological abuse on the emotional well-being and quality of life of adult survivors.

Despite the significant challenges posed by child psychological abuse, there is hope for adult survivors. Research on the human brain provides a glimmer of hope for individuals who have experienced this type of trauma. It suggests that the synapses and neural pathways in the brain are remarkably adaptable and capable of creating alternative routes to achieve new goals and functions (Baker & Schneiderman, 2015). For instance, if one part of the brain suffers damage, another part may compensate and regain functionality with the appropriate support (Baker & Schneiderman, 2015). This implies that survivors of abuse are not condemned to forever enact a predetermined blueprint of behaviour and maladaptive beliefs if they choose to embark on a journey of healing and growth (Baker & Schneiderman, 2015).

However, the formation of early ideas about oneself and the surrounding world, such as feeling stupid, unworthy, or bad, can be deeply ingrained and challenging to alter (Baker & Schneiderman, 2015). These ideas become woven into the foundation view and core schemas about the world and oneself, shaping perceptions and behaviours in adulthood (Baker & Schneiderman, 2015).

Moreover, the Researcher is currently developing a treatment framework outlined in Volume Three. This framework aims to harness the brain's neuroplasticity to facilitate changes in neural pathways and belief systems. Through the new ideas presented, survivors and their MHPs will be guided in exploring and addressing deep-seated emotional wounds and distorted perceptions formed during infancy (Baker & Schneiderman, 2015). By providing a safe and supportive environment for self-reflection and transformation, the framework seeks to empower survivors to rewrite their core narratives and cultivate healthier perspectives on themselves and the world around them.

The crucial role of early caregiver-infant relationships in shaping lifelong biobehavioral regulation, including the reactivity of the hypothalamus-pituitary-adrenal (HPA) axis, underscores the importance of interventions aimed at fostering supportive environments for healing and growth among adult survivors of parental alienation and child psychological abuse.

For example, the "quality of the relationship between infants and caregivers during stages of early brain development seems to be a critical determinant of lifelong biobehavioral regulation, including hypothalamus-pituitary-adrenal (HPA) axis reactivity, in the offspring" (Carpenter et al., 2009, p. 69). If the 'good enough parent' regulates her and the infant's autonomic nervous system sufficiently, this will moderate the infant's experience of extreme high and low arousal (Winnicott, 1960). However, when maltreatment or relational trauma is present, the caregiver either actively overstimulates the infant through frightening behaviour and abuse or under-stimulated through neglect (Alexander, 2015). Either way, the caregiver fails to protect the infant from stress and danger, and through their inaccessibility, they fail to regulate the infant's over or under-arousal response (Winnicott, n.d).

The study conducted by Carpenter et al. (2009, p.69) underscores the reactivity of the hypothalamus-pituitary-adrenal (HPA) axis as a potential indicator of susceptibility to various stress-related diseases and neuropsychiatric disorders. Adults with a history of maltreatment often experience an amplification of the effects of childhood abuse as they age, indicating a cumulative response to their early-life adversity (Carpenter et al., 2009).

Moreover, acute psychosocial stress, characterised by both exaggerated and blunted cortisol responses or neuroendocrine challenges, has been strongly associated with disease in humans (Carpenter et al., 2009). Exposure to stress, particularly in the form of emotional abuse during critical developmental periods in childhood, can have enduring effects on both behavioural and physiological aspects throughout an individual's life, potentially increasing their susceptibility to stress-related diseases (Carpenter et al., 2009).

Emotional abuse, if experienced persistently for a decade or more during childhood, can become a chronic stressor, leading to difficulties in interpersonal relationships and attachment, thus perpetuating chronic stress in the adult child's relationships across their life (Carpenter et al., 2009).

Emotional Manipulation Leading to Brain Washing

Examining additional dimensions of emotional manipulation, prior studies concerning adult survivors of PA reveal exposure to various "emotional manipulation strategies" (Baker, 2007, p. 12). These strategies include withdrawing love, fostering dependency, and establishing loyalty binds by the alienating parents (Baker, 2007). The adult survivors also described their APs as using brainwashing techniques in the form of "repetitive negative statements" regarding their targeted parent (TP) as well as black-and-white thinking (Baker, 2007, p. 32). Early research describes this phenomenon as "the cult of parenthood" and reports that brainwashing or programming children is a key component of PA (Baker, 2007, pp. 32, 84).

The Similarity between Cults and SPA

Bridging the gap between these findings and broader academic perspectives, previous researchers have studied brainwashing and thought reform within neuroscience and social psychology (Taylor, 2017). They studied cult members from small-scale cults, such as Charles Manson' who created the 'Manson Family' to larger-scale cults, such as the Reverend Jim Jones (The Jonestown Massacre), who operated in the isolated jungle area of Guyana (Taylor, 2017).

In Taylor's (2017, p. xiii) book, brainwashing is delineated into three approaches aimed at altering individuals' beliefs: through force, stealth, and direct brain manipulation techniques. Cults typically employ strategies such as isolating victims from their previous environments, controlling their perceptions, thoughts, and actions, inducing uncertainty about prior beliefs, instilling new beliefs through repetition, and manipulating emotions to weaken old beliefs and reinforce new ones (Taylor, 2017, p. xiii).

This framework resonates with the dynamics observed in cases of SPA, where children may have been abducted and isolated from one parent, controlled in their perceptions and behaviour, induced to doubt their previous beliefs, subjected to repeated reinforcement of new beliefs, and emotionally manipulated. These findings from Taylor's (2017) analysis not only corroborate earlier research on PA but also align with the reported experiences of adult survivors in this study, further emphasising the pervasive use of brainwashing within PA contexts.

Tactics Used to Brainwash the Adult Survivor as a Child

Early research conducted by Baker (2007) identifies five primary manipulation techniques utilised to persuade, control, and manipulate children within cases of PA. These techniques include relentlessly denigrating or bad-mouthing the character of the targeted parent, fostering a narrative that portrays the targeted parent as dangerous and intending to harm the child, misrepresenting the targeted parent's feelings toward the child to fostering resentment and psychological distance, withholding love from the child when they express positive regard or affection for the TP, and minimising both actual and symbolic contact with the TP, effectively erasing them from the child's life and psyche (Baker, 2007, p. 84).

Psychiatrist Dr. Robert Jay Lifton (1969) describes these five brainwashing techniques as consistent with thought reform methods (Baker, 2007). These techniques generate psychological stimuli in the environment that reach the individual's inner emotions. This observation aligns with the distinctions made by Clawar and Rivlan (1991) between programming and brainwashing. Programming refers to the substance of the message, while brainwashing refers to the actions employed to communicate these messages (Baker, 2007).

In cases of PA, the AP operates under the belief that by repeatedly exposing their child to a certain narrative, it will eventually become accepted as truth by the child (Clawar & Rivlin, 2014). When Baker's research was published in 2007, it highlighted a lack of information regarding how and when adult survivors disengage from the "cult of parenthood" (Baker, 2007, p. 167). In the absence of sufficient data on children of PA, Baker drew parallels with research on former cult members. These individuals reported leaving the group either voluntarily, being expelled, or as a result of counselling (Baker, 2007).

This exploration sets the stage for understanding Bowlby's groundbreaking concept developed in 1958. Bowlby presented a pioneering concept that outlined the connection between the brain and heart of individuals who undergo successful brainwashing and coercion and the relationship between the leader and follower (Stein, 2021). While fear is commonly associated with fleeing from something, Bowlby (1958) suggests that individuals also tend to seek comfort and support from another person (Stein, 2021). In the context of child psychological abuse, the AP assumes the role of a safe haven towards which children of PA gravitate when they are afraid. This manipulation occurs through isolating the child from other potential sources of comfort, inducing fear in them (Stein, 2021). However, this behaviour does not reflect a healthy means of seeking protection when frightened; rather, it represents a hard-wired, problematic behaviour known as a disorganised attachment (Stein, 2021).

Disorganised attachment in children of PA arises when the child encounters frightening situations without a clear solution. Typically, the child instinctively seeks comfort from the caregiver. However, in cases of SPA, the caregiver serves as both the source of safety and the cause of distress (Stein, 2021). This contradictory role creates an impossible situation for the child, leading to the collapse of their attachment strategies and a sense of disorganisation.

Consequently, the child may oscillate between approaching the frightening parent (the AP) and attempting to avoid fearful stimuli from them. This conflicting behaviour often manifests as confusion, freezing, and a range of other behaviours (Stein, 2021). "The child may exhibit rapid shifts between seeking proximity to the AP and withdrawing from them" (Stein, 2021, p. 39). Despite the desire to escape the fear-inducing AP, the child's innate need for closeness typically prevails, resulting in their continued proximity to the frightening caregiver.

This complex dynamic underscores the profound challenges faced by children of child psychological abuse linked to SPA, with implications extending into adulthood. This difficult state has been reported in this research, supporting this volume within 80% of the adult survivors of SPA. This discovery is another indication that a treatment protocol for MHPs to use with survivors needs to be developed.

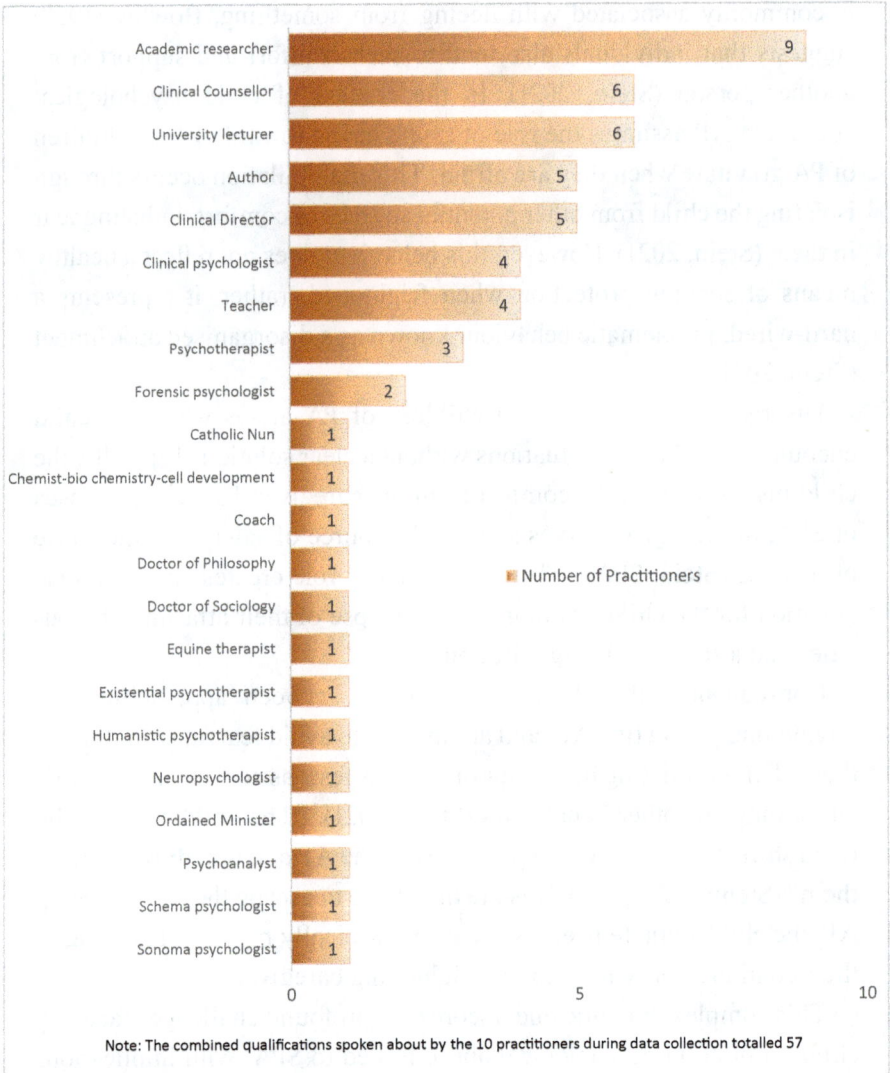

Qualification	Number of Practitioners
Academic researcher	9
Clinical Counsellor	6
University lecturer	6
Author	5
Clinical Director	5
Clinical psychologist	4
Teacher	4
Psychotherapist	3
Forensic psychologist	2
Catholic Nun	1
Chemist-bio chemistry-cell development	1
Coach	1
Doctor of Philosophy	1
Doctor of Sociology	1
Equine therapist	1
Existential psychotherapist	1
Humanistic psychotherapist	1
Neuropsychologist	1
Ordained Minister	1
Psychoanalyst	1
Schema psychologist	1
Sonoma psychologist	1

Note: The combined qualifications spoken about by the 10 practitioners during data collection totalled 57

FIGURE EIGHT

Combined Qualifications of Mental Health Practitioners

Specialty Areas Practised by Mental Health Practitioners

The kaleidoscope of specialty areas practised among the ten MHPs ranged from complex family matters and trauma, research, university lecturing, cults, abduction, kidnapping, paternity fraud, familicide, child abuse assessment and more, as presented in Figure Nine. Interestingly,

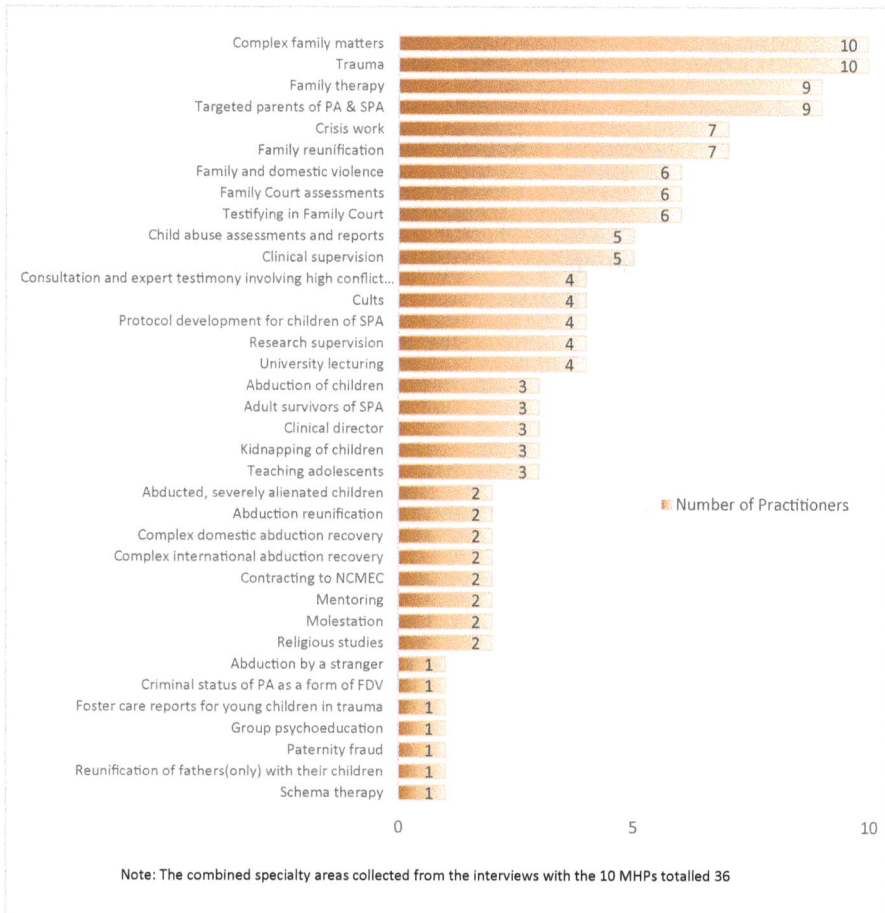

Specialty Area	Number of Practitioners
Complex family matters	10
Trauma	10
Family therapy	9
Targeted parents of PA & SPA	9
Crisis work	7
Family reunification	7
Family and domestic violence	6
Family Court assessments	6
Testifying in Family Court	6
Child abuse assessments and reports	5
Clinical supervision	5
Consultation and expert testimony involving high conflict...	4
Cults	4
Protocol development for children of SPA	4
Research supervision	4
University lecturing	4
Abduction of children	3
Adult survivors of SPA	3
Clinical director	3
Kidnapping of children	3
Teaching adolescents	3
Abducted, severely alienated children	2
Abduction reunification	2
Complex domestic abduction recovery	2
Complex international abduction recovery	2
Contracting to NCMEC	2
Mentoring	2
Molestation	2
Religious studies	2
Abduction by a stranger	1
Criminal status of PA as a form of FDV	1
Foster care reports for young children in trauma	1
Group psychoeducation	1
Paternity fraud	1
Reunification of fathers(only) with their children	1
Schema therapy	1

Note: The combined specialty areas collected from the interviews with the 10 MHPs totalled 36

FIGURE NINE

Specialty Areas Practised by Mental Health Practitioners

all MHPs worked in areas linked to the different dynamics within a family structure. The combined speciality areas collected from the data totalled thirty-six.

Backgrounds of the Mental Health Practitioners

MHPs with a minimum of a bachelor's degree or postgraduate degree in psychology or psychotherapy who work clinically with survivors were interviewed for these studies using semi-structured interviews. Within this subtheme, data were reported from MHPs working in clinical and professional settings, including private practice, family reunification, Family Court, homeless organisations, prisons and youth detention centres, mental health units and Children's Courts. The combined number of MHPs reported qualifications totalled fifty-seven. MHPs cited qualifications in more than one specialty area or profession. The combined years of the study participants' professional experience working in the mental health sector totalled two hundred and sixty-seven based on years of experience reported during data collection.

Practitioner's Country of Origin and Gender

MHPs were recruited from Australia (4), The United Kingdom (1), Canada (2), and The United States of America (3). These practitioners were identified by the social constructionist genders of four males and six females (Wamsley, 2021), and they were between thirty-five and eighty-two years old (Wamsley, 2021). Nine participants identified as 'white', and one identified as 'African-American'.

Therapists with Lived Experience (TLE)

Within this sub-theme, the term 'therapist with lived experience' (TLE) describes therapists with lived personal experience of mental health challenges who are professionally recognised as registered counsellors, psychotherapists, psychologists, or other trained therapists (The ATLEN, 2017). Among the ten practitioners, two identified as survivors of PA. A third practitioner identified as an adult survivor of SPA and participated in both the adult survivor and MHP interviews.

Additionally, five of the ten MHPs in the study self-identified as TLEs and referenced this topic twenty-nine times within the coded data. The discovery of therapists identifying as TLEs in the data was an exciting finding. As explained in MHP Chapter Six, MHPs who identify as TLEs are often stigmatised within their collegial groups (Cooper et al., 2020). The fact that 50% of the MHP study participants identified as TLEs prompts the Researcher to question if the current low numbers of identification among this cohort are correct or if this figure of 50% is an accurate reflection of the mental health sector, but the TLE MHPs are not feeling safe enough to disclose.

Trauma research suggests that TLEs must have the choice to safely disclose (The ATLEN, 2017). Moving through trauma when working professionally with clients who are experiencing suicidality or trauma that the therapist themselves may have experienced, such as the extracts provided by the study participants, can be undertaken with the proper supervision and private counselling. For example, experienced TLEs practise the skill of bracketing to help them manage conflicts about personal values and stop them from imposing their values onto clients (McWhorter, 2019). Bracketing allows TLEs to revisit their emotional reactions after being triggered in a session on their own time and again during clinical supervision or private counselling.

TLEs offer two lenses rather than only one from which to look through when working with clients and provide best-practice interventions in accordance with their professional training (The ATLEN, 2017). TLEs claim to be empowered and cognisant of the service-user movement's human rights and recovery perceptions (The ATLEN, 2017). Study data captured from the TLE MHPs emerged from sharing their own trauma experiences. Positions constructed from MHPs varied, ranging from 40% of TLEs openly self-identifying and 10% not wanting it known that they have lived experience themselves, nor do they wish to integrate the patient and therapist identity.

Earlier studies suggest that the challenge of merging the identities of patients and therapists is significantly impacted by the societal perceptions associated with the therapist and patient roles, which often create a sense of separation between the two (Cleary & Armour, 2022). The following paragraph exemplifies a current real-life "them and us dynamic" (Cleary & Armour, 2022, p. 1100). This example occurred when the Researcher spoke to her colleague, 'RUOK Ambassador' and lived experience speaker, Mr Glenn Cotter. Permission was obtained to use his name and to add the 'them and us' perspective recount on TLEs, disclosure and telling clients about being a TLE when they are experiencing suicidal ideation or have made a suicide attempt. Mr Cotter was invited to speak as a guest lecturer to undergraduate psychology students at The University of Wollongong (UOW). Mr Cotter spoke to the psychology students about potentially identifying as TLEs after graduation. Mr Cotter shared his learnings from this engagement with the Researcher for these studies in the following extract;

> Many of the students in the lecture put their hands up when I asked if they had lived experience of attempted suicide or suicidal ideation. However, when I asked them later if they would identify as a psychologist with lived experience to their potential clients when they graduate, they said no. There is a paradox between 'them and us' that I see as someone employed as a lived experience suicide support worker. It seems taboo for psychologists to admit they have lived experience, yet my clients openly state that they want their therapists to have lived experience, not just a university degree. So, what will the psychologists say when a client asks if they have lived experience of a suicide attempt by someone who is suicidal? If they don't have experience, they'll be

discussing a topic they don't truly understand. If they admit they don't have experience, the client may never return. However, I can answer that truthfully because I understand the space between suicidal ideation and an attempt. Maybe by sharing, I will save someone's life. (G. Cotter, personal communication, January 13th, 2023)

The interview information that Mr Cotter shared regarding practitioners not wanting to disclose was replicated within this research by one MHP. As a reminder, 40% of MHPs said they would reveal they were a TLE, 10% did not want the client to know, and 50% did not answer. This data is a notable finding considering that previous research reports that MHPs may not disclose being a TLE due to experiencing trepidation and concerns that their perceived competency may be scrutinised when working in organisational cultures of non-disclosure (Cleary & Armour, 2022). These studies report that the MHPs were highly experienced in trauma and consequently felt more secure in their abilities. Thereby, sharing their own lived experience was a way to work with clients who felt suicidal and connect on a deeper level when appropriate, despite how they were advised by governing bodies.

The data also showed that survivors of suicidal ideation or who have attempted suicide would request a TLE to work with them instead of an MHP without experience of this kind. For example, three of the eleven adult child survivors who participated in this research had explicitly requested an MHP with lived experience of suicidal ideation due to PA or SPA when looking for therapy. These study participants' results report that TLEs can be therapists of other lived experiences, not just suicide attempts or ideation. MHP participants in these studies who identify as TLEs described examples of their mental and physical experiences during data collection.

For example, some MHP experiences encompassed PA, SPA, sexual assault, FDV and IPV in their marriages. One MHP participant positioned themselves as a survivor of a failed abortion attempt by their mother. Another practitioner positioned themselves as a child of PA. Finally, a fifth practitioner self-identified as 'the Golden Child' in their family and a 'regulatory object for their mother' but did not feel they were a child of PA and did not describe themselves as a TLE. However, during the interview, the Researcher noted that this participant understood the dynamics of PA from a child's perspective and explained that this was why they specialised in this field. Results gleaned from this research report show that practitioners who identify as TLEs are not limited to talking about their suicide attempts or ideation but branch out to include other life experiences that they are willing to speak about if they deem it helpful and pertinent to the client at the time.

Family Reunification Practitioners

Four MHPs in these studies specialise in family reunification; three of the four participants are also TLEs. The third practitioner specialises in reuniting children under 18 with their biological fathers. This practitioner adopts various measures, including DNA testing, retaining attorneys, engaging therapists, and employing private investigators to locate missing, alienated children.

The fourth participant explained that they have worked with about 20 family reunifications, including first reunifications, holidays, residence transfers, and international abduction cases. This MHP also shared that they are a TLE and a TP who has personally experienced FDV. The violence they experienced encompassed both burglary and sexual abuse perpetrated by their former partner within the confines of their own home. This practitioner shared that they stopped seeing their alienated children on a therapist's advice to safeguard them. Instead, this practitioner constructed their understanding and meaning of what was happening in their life by educating themselves and searching on social media for information about their children.

Additionally, the MHP they engaged for themselves for their own counselling did not provide any construction of meaning or interpretation of PA and SPA during the time of the abuse. However, this MHP independently acquired knowledge about their situation, including the terminology of 'parental alienation', through self-education on the Internet, interestingly mirroring the survivors' self-learnings. This lived experience has consequently led the practitioner to specialise in family reunification.

Reasons for Working in the Field of Parental Alienation

In constructing the MHPs' experiences of why they work in the field of SPA, one of the study participants explained that they were intrigued by the family dynamics in SPA and felt the need to make sense of the chaos they saw. However, this practitioner also explained that working in the trauma field with the associated family and social systems was problematic due to their lack of specific training;

> I realised other practitioners didn't want to stay in the room with these sorts of issues. And I found them intriguing to work with. It's intriguing how to sit in the middle of that kind of chaotic, difficult family system. And so, when I went back and trained as a family therapist because up until that time, I've been working more as an individual therapist, it all started to make sense. So, while I knew about systems theory and Bronfenbrenner, his approach to looking at people, they're always in different social systems, etc. When I did the family therapy training, and they were looking at some of the key concepts about how families with boundary issues, you know, they act in particular ways, and then I was starting to know, ah, that's what it is. (MHP8)

In this extract, MHP8 talks about how their role as a practitioner is problematised by seeing the other practitioners not wanting to work with this complex client group even though she found them intriguing. This practitioner constructs a lack of training in the field as an area for professional development and positions herself as presenting a solution, leading her to specialise in this area. This notion follows from the tradition of social constructionism created by Mead (1930) regarding the concept of "symbolic interactionism", which argues that human beings can construct their own identities through everyday encounters and social interactions with others (Mead, 1934, p. 112). Other study participants also emphasised this concept within the transcripts. They shared that developing an understanding of survivors and their trauma was also problematised by a lack of specific training to identify survivors of PA and SPA.

Number of SPA Cases MHP has Worked With Professionally

This next topic presents results regarding how many survivors' participants had worked professionally. The answers ranged from "just a few because they generally don't present to therapy" (MHP1), "probably a few cases" (MHP's 2 and 7), "fifteen" (MHP5), "forty to fifty" (MHP4), "hundreds" (MHP8), "50% of the cases" (MHP6), "I'm not a fan of the professional diagnosis names. They're too labelling and take away the humanness" (MHP10), and "89% of the cases, or about 300 plus" (MHP9).

In addition, participants described their therapeutic work with the survivors as made challenging by the "sheer number of people sent to them for assessment" (MHP7). Numerous participants constructed their understanding of the number of survivors they encountered as requesting therapeutic work. Some of these accounts formed the experience of survivors as problematic due to SPA's differing social dimensions not being considered, leading to practitioners not noticing the underlying symptoms, especially when survivors present with disguised presentations (Gelinas, 1983).

One study participant expressed concern over other MHPs not being knowledgeable enough regarding survivors' challenges. MHP1 positioned themselves as aware of the other practitioners' professional challenges by describing, "Still, no one is treating the underlying issues. The contemplative nature of survivors is due to not realising what is going on with their mental health, drug, and alcohol abuse issues, and only being treated for the presenting issues". MHP1 explained their position on presenting survivors and their treating MHPs;

> The second group – the more severe group – have mental health issues: depression, substance abuse, all sorts – but they're getting treated for all of that, and nobody's identifying the underlying family attachment issues or social impact going on. So this could be an extremely widespread pathology; it's just that no one's diagnosing it. They don't present; that's a very rare population to present to therapy. And there's a spectrum of the population. A lot of them are pretty contemplative; they're not realising what's going on, and they're just starting to become aware. They're diagnosing the substance abuse. They're diagnosing the suicide attempts. They're diagnosing depression– they're diagnosing everything around it except the attachment pathology. And that's where you go with severe parental alienation. I will translate that over into severe attachment pathology. (MHP1)

In this previous extract, MHP1 explains that their role as a clinical psychologist is being problematised by the widespread pathology of SPA and believes that other practitioners are only diagnosing SPA symptoms and not the root cause. This practitioner also shared that other MHPs may only be seeing survivors presenting with mild to moderate PA and not the severe range of symptoms that go along with the broader social aspect of SPA due to survivors not realising what is going on for them. Finally, MHP1 states that many other MHPs do not understand the attachment pathology or the effect of the social impact that survivors may still be experiencing.

The Broader Social Impact of PA and SPA

The following TLE MHP constructs an offshoot of SPA's broader social impact, CITs and effects on survivors who have been 'cut off' from a parent and the broader community. This practitioner also positions themselves as not agreeing that the term PA or SPA fully addresses the complexity of alienation and the other social dimensions that a survivor may have encountered;

> I would suggest that the vast majority of people I worked with in agencies over the past 22 years have had mild PA experiences. For me, really severe, that's only been maybe half a dozen people. I would think that it's been so significant that the cut-off has been permanent, not a bit. The cut-off isn't just from the parent. It extends into the broader community and name changes and things like that. Severe has a broader impact. My trauma work with adults has been very complex trauma family, non-familial abduction, familial abduction, and captivity. People held them captive. And so if it's a family-based, they know pretty clearly, but in some ways, I think it's even better because they're like, No, I was abducted and held captive by my parents. You call it parental alienation that doesn't even touch it. (ID withheld for confidentiality)

The data collected from this deidentified TLE MHP differed significantly from the other study participants in that this practitioner has specialised in SPA, with the added CITs of children and adults who have also been abducted, tortured, and held captive. This practitioner is part of a small group of specialists who collaborate closely and from whom they construct their professional knowledge. This practitioner believes they have only seen six genuine SPA cases in their extensive career. This practitioner also shared that the police will not get involved in family court matters nor return a child whom an AP has abducted. This MHP does not believe that the term 'severe parental alienation' comes close to identifying this phenomenon's broad social impact and complex nature. One of the suggestions made by the Researcher regarding a different name for children of abduction was not to call children or adults victims of SPA but victims of 'SPAA'.

During data collection, this practitioner openly stated that they were part of a small group of specialist SPA practitioners. Therefore, data were collected from the other study participants to understand collegial support levels for specialist practitioners within the SPA field and presented in the following subtheme.

Number of Therapists Known to MHPs Working in PA and SPA

The MHPs were asked how many other practitioners they know who work with survivors. Five practitioners responded, and their answers contained a number with an additional comment. The first practitioner, 'MHP4', answered, "About twenty or thirty. I know a lot who don't know what they're doing. But I also work with people who know what they're doing". The second practitioner, 'MHP3', explained, "I run a practice in Australia that employs twenty-five clinical and forensic psychologists, but none specialise in PA or SPA. This could be because I haven't been 'tuning in' either". The third practitioner, 'MHP7', answered, "A small number throughout the United States", and a fourth practitioner, 'MHP5', answered, "Zero, none in America". Finally, the fifth practitioner, 'MHP2', explained that he knows a few practitioners who work with survivors. He added that his knowledge was constructed from a handful of previous research on PA and SPA that his colleagues had undertaken before him:

I have amongst my colleagues the people I look up to. I look up to them as the people who made me understand the work that I'm doing. They have researched, they've theorised about it, and they understand what it is and how it manifests. Only one of them is a sociologist. All the rest are clinical psychologists. There are very few social workers, very few counsellors/psychotherapists, and so they understand it within a narrow silo. (MHP2)

Half of the MHPs in these studies highlighted a lack of experienced MHP colleagues in the field of PA and SPA. However, as the MHPs constructed their own experiences, they shared that they were aware of colleagues they believed knew what they were doing versus those who did not within this small group, and they surmised that there was a limited pool from which to draw knowledge. MHP knowledge was constructed from learnings from other colleagues and previous research.

Summary

This part of the chapter has reported on participant data, such as practitioner backgrounds, qualifications, specialist areas, training recommendations, and the social impact on survivors and TLEs. Study participants responded to the worldwide recruitment request, making it a global study that adds real-world data to the dearth of available information on survivors. The background data collected on the MHPs reported that 50% of the participants identified as survivors of PA, 10% as survivors of SPA, 20% as TP, and 10% had experienced IPV and FDV. Of note was the high number of specialty areas in the cohort. This high number reflected the amount of extensive academic experience within the group, with 90% of the participants describing themselves as having experience as a Researcher, followed by 60% stating two separate professional job descriptions- clinical counsellor and university lecturer.

Of note were the findings from 50% of the participants who reported on colleagues who therapeutically treat survivors. These numbers differed significantly. For example, 20% reported knowing no one or a small group, and 10% reported working with over 20 clinical psychologists. However, 20% specialised in child and adult survivors of SPA, and a further 20% stated that 50% of the practitioners they identified did not know what they were doing. This finding was notable, considering that research suggests that approximately 4.3 million children are estimated to be moderately to severely alienated from their TP in America (Harman et al., 2019). In the following Theme One, study participants report their perspectives regarding the training and development they consider fundamental to working in the SPA field. In addition, the CITs reported to practitioners by survivors are reported upon within the sub-themes.

KEY THEME ONE

SPA Complex Intersecting Trauma (CIT) Reported to MHPs

The data corpus was examined using a social constructionist thematic analysis (Braun & Clarke, 2014). Three main superordinate themes emerged from the MHPs' data. Theme One: SPA Complex Intersecting Traumas and Sub Themes reported to the MHPs by survivors. Theme Two: A sample of the modalities, therapies and perspectives of MHPs when treating survivors. Finally, Theme Three: A sample of professional training and development recommendations.

Theme One highlights the constraints, challenges, broader social dimensions, and impacts MHPs experience. For example, study participants reported the lack of specific SPA training and development and the absence of direction regarding treatment options to use with survivors. Also reported was the kaleidoscope of CITs and social dimensions that survivors speak to practitioners about during therapy. The following paragraphs address some of the CITs gleaned from the participant data that MHPs outside of these studies must be aware of when embarking on therapy with survivors.

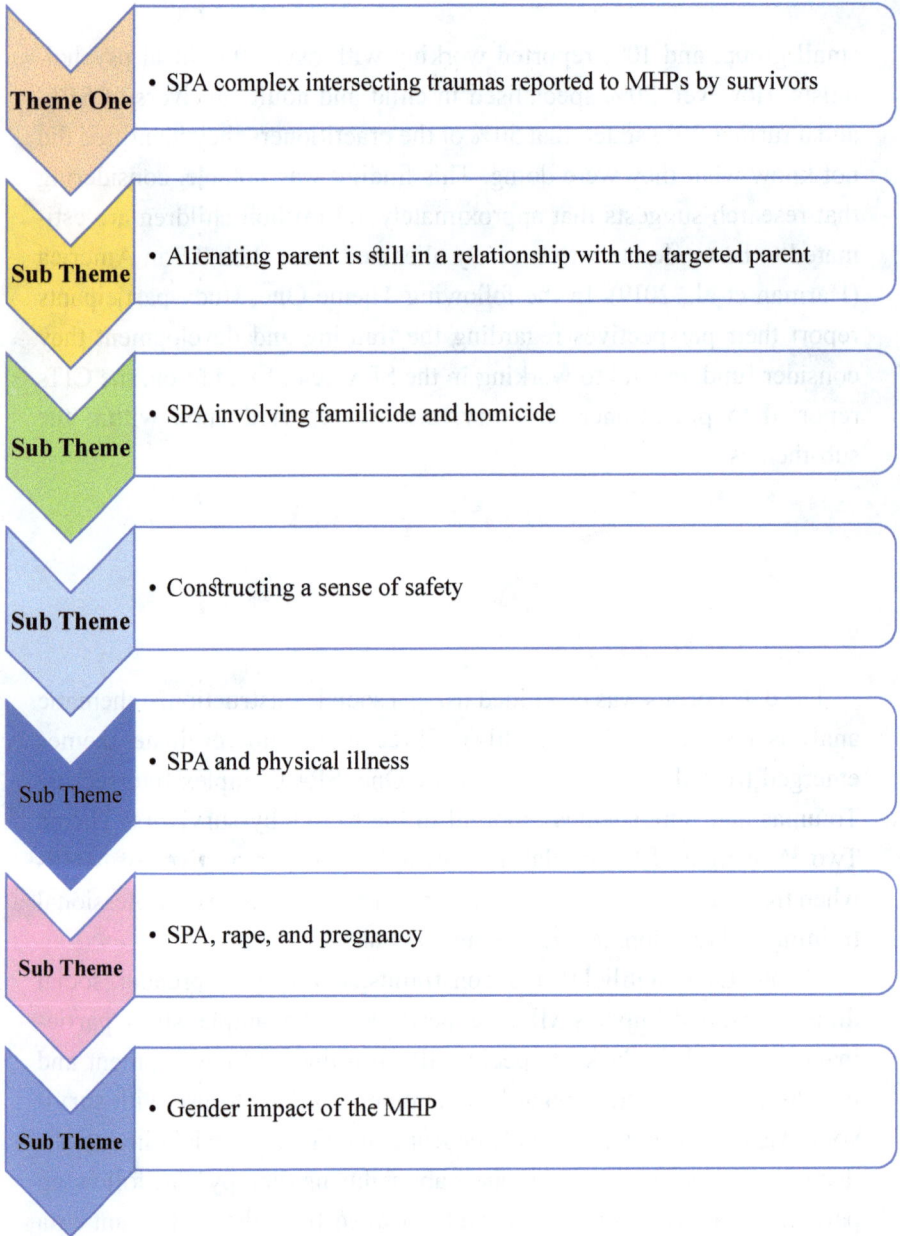

Theme One	• SPA complex intersecting traumas reported to MHPs by survivors
Sub Theme	• Alienating parent is still in a relationship with the targeted parent
Sub Theme	• SPA involving familicide and homicide
Sub Theme	• Constructing a sense of safety
Sub Theme	• SPA and physical illness
Sub Theme	• SPA, rape, and pregnancy
Sub Theme	• Gender impact of the MHP

FIGURE TEN

Main Theme One and Sub Themes from Data Collected from MHPs

Alienating Parents are Still Together

Within the following subthemes, one MHP reported the construction of SPA CITs experienced by survivors. This practitioner explained that PA and SPA might be an active family dynamic within intact families, not just families that have experienced separation and divorce. The term family dynamics pertains to the highly individual workings within a family. Dynamics, including overt and covert mannerisms, can be expressed directly and indirectly (Gerhardt, 2019). Each family is unique, and different family dynamics will influence particular views of family members about themselves and their world (Gerhardt, 2019). The following extract is an example shared by MHP8, which constructed their therapeutic work with survivors as made challenging due to the intricate family dynamics that are playing out among the older siblings of the presenting client;

> This is an unusual situation because the parents are still together, but they alienate. They actually use the partner as the regulatory object. When they get together, then the children are born. And now, the children are the regulatory objects. And as long as the partner is still enmeshed with them, everything's okay. My client's the regulatory object for the whole family. And so the other sisters, one has gone completely wild, one's on drugs, alcohol, multiple substances, multiple partners, can't be in a relationship. That's the eldest sister, the next sister down. She's chaotic in behaviour. When she's regulated, life is good for her other sister, which is my client; when her sister is not regulated, then that gets really tricky. My client presented with a relational difficulty, but we finally talked about family and domestic violence after probably about a year of working together. (MHP8)

In this extract, MHP8 talks about their role as a clinical psychologist being problematised by the complex family dynamics in an intact family during family therapy sessions. MHP8 also reports that the adult survivor of SPA initially presented in session with issues about relational difficulties, but it was a year before they spoke about the FDV they were experiencing. FDV is defined as "any behaviour that's violent, threatening, controlling or intended to make you or your family feel scared and unsafe" (Australian Government, 2022, p. 1). This behaviour can evolve into a more sinister form of violence and is a complex intersecting trauma (CIT) that MHPs must be alert for when working with an adult survivor.

Familicide and Homicide

Familicide

This next, more serious level of CIT is known as familicide and homicide. The term familicide has been employed to encompass diverse forms of homicide within families (Karlsson et al., 2021). Familicide involves a perpetrator intentionally killing or attempting to kill their current or former partner and one or more of their biological children or stepchildren (Karlsson et al., 2021). Additionally, previous research reports that a divorce or separation precedes the majority of familicide occurrences and that firearms are the most frequently utilised method of murder. The adult female partner is typically presumed to be the main target of the offender, with the children being killed because the perpetrator views them as an extension of their partner (Karlsson et al., 2021).

Familicides frequently emerge as a secondary topic in studies that have wider research objectives, such as examining homicide-suicide or offender populations with mental health issues. As a result, only a subset of familicide incidents may be incorporated. Details about familicide may be merged with data about other homicides, making it difficult to distinguish specific information about familicide (Karlsson et al., 2021). This is a point that MHPs need to consider when a survivor presents for therapy. Familicide is another CIT of SPA reported within this research data. An example is offered in the following paragraph.

Four MHPs in the study reported working with the complex issue of familicide and homicide among survivors of SPA. MHP8 explained that one social dimension of SPA is a form of FDV, which can occur when the parents fight so much that one parent decides to kill the children. Another example given by a different study participant was reported as a 'SPA and familicide case' where one person was immobilised by their partner, shooting them in the hip and then went on to murder both their children. According to MHP8, "MHPs may face this CIT when working with children and survivors, as killing children or threatening to kill them is a common threat to children of SPA". However, MHP8 also added that "familicide is something that the alienating parent would be likelier to do than the targeted parent".

Abduction and Threats of Being Killed

Constructing a sense of safety for the client is a complex issue that MHPs may face if they work with survivors of SPA who have been abducted and had threats of being killed by a parent. One MHP explained (ID withheld for confidentiality);

> When the (agency withheld) has called me, there were two children taken to a different country, and they believe their mother had stopped looking, and I had the (withheld) bring the flier and a (withheld) bring the missing cancelled checks to show them that, indeed, this was not the right story. So, you must stop this shit as soon as possible. This bullshit of always showing pictures of the family being happy it's just a crock of shit that can't help, but that's not it. You have to be really mindful, authentic, and purposeful and hit it right out of the gate and say, look, your father's not trying to kill you. He never tried to kill you. One of the things we know from the (agency withheld) is the parent that usually, the parent who's been left behind would never take the children from the other parent. (ID withheld for confidentiality)

MHPs may also need to construct a sense of safety for themselves, especially concerning preventing vicarious trauma in PA and SPA. For example, MHP (ID withheld for confidentiality) also shared that working with clients involved with abduction, homicide detectives, and forensic police attracts people who attack them and make board complaints against them, not allowing them to feel safe when they work. For readers who have perused the preceding two paragraphs, it may be inferred that the occurrence of familicide and abduction represents a traumatic experience for children and adults who have experienced SPA. However, the following subtheme examines another concern for MHPs when working with survivors: the threat of physical illness due to SPA trauma for survivors.

SPA and Physical Illness Among Adult Survivors

During the interviews, MHPs were asked about their biggest concerns when working with survivors. As a result, two participants shared about the physical illness side of SPA and the symptom severity they see in their clients;

> Oh, God, it's the physical illnesses that they've developed as a result of carrying it in their body the load. A few months ago, I just started seeing a young woman 14, she just turned 14, and she's been diagnosed with cancer. She came because she thought she was anxious about cancer. Her history is horrible. And severe alienation is all over it. And for me, it's finding strength within me to help carry some of that burden and damage and to help them process their reactions to what happens in their relationship. The hardest part for me is helping them come to terms with the gravity of what happened to them. (MHP4)

In this extract, the damaging effects of abuse are constructed as a consequence of the client's body carrying the trauma load. This practitioner assumes a position that is an intuitive, caring, feminine approach composed in a way where they deliberately choose to internally carry some of the burdens for the adult survivors themselves, hoping to allow their clients to make sense of the abuse they have experienced. Alongside this position, the effects of SPA abuse were constructed by the practitioner as the consequence of faulty catastrophic associations and connections that subsequently lead to the manifestation of distressing symptoms becoming a reality through the onset of a serious physical illness. Jones (1991) emphasises the relevance of considering a practitioner's gender within the therapeutic relationship and how this could affect their subsequent work (Jones, 1991). Both draw from the feminist approaches of considering the power relations between gender differences and the broader socio-political framework that privileges males over females.

SPA, Rape and Gender

Herman (1998) reports on the importance of contemplating gender differences between clients and their MHPs when a survivor has experienced rape. Of note is the influence on how male practitioners may position themselves when working with a female SPA client, emphasising potential professional consequences in this context and the inclusion of boundary violations. This concept constructs recovery as potentially occurring within a therapeutic relationship that may experience potential transference and countertransference experiences. However, gender as a factor when working with survivors of SPA and rape must be considered sensitively by the treating practitioner.

For male or non-binary MHPs, this topic may require additional professional support during clinical supervision to address any projection or countertransference they may experience. Likewise, additional clinical supervision may also need to be implemented for female practitioners who may experience transference or countertransference from survivors who have experienced sexual abuse or rape, especially when the practitioner may have been raped. In these cases, extra clinical supervision when working with clients with whom they share a similar trauma experience is important to prevent countertransference and vicarious trauma. Finally, rape is not just something that happens to girls or women. MHPs, no matter their gender, may have experienced rape.

SPA and Pregnancy Due to Rape

According to TLE MHP5, who identifies as an African-American female working to stop the continuing intergenerational 'fatherless generations,' SPA is a widespread problem in her community. This MHP describes the complexity and CITs in the following extract that she faces when working with clients who have experienced SPA and rape within her community. TLE MHP5 shares the events that have led this client (a young African-American mother) to work with her and how as a practitioner, she positions herself as needing to help not only the mother who was raped and also did not know she was an adult survivor of SPA and adoption but also her twin girls who will grow up without a father;

> She didn't even know that she had an alienation problem. She's a single mom wanting to get around the trauma because she has twin girls due to rape. And so she was like, 'they're not going to have a father. They're just not!'. So how do we help them be better? They're not going to be perfect. But how do we help them be the best possible young ladies that they can be? So, I was giving her tools. A year and a half later, she finds out she's adopted. And that's why her mother treated her so badly. And as she goes through that journey, she realises this is why I'm married to men who were fatherless. What if they had someone who helped them identify the trauma, the childhood trauma from their fatherless journey? Walk them through a healing process. The point is you've got to heal your childhood trauma. TLE (MHP5)

TLE MHP5 describes an experience within her community where fathers are absent and not deemed necessary to rearing children, especially after being conceived by rape. Rape and sexual abuse are also constructed as a consequence of another person 'going too far.'

This chapter section has reported on subthemes collected from the participants, such as intact families experiencing alienation, constructing a sense of safety for survivors during a session, the links between SPA and physical illness reported by survivors to practitioners, SPA, rape, and gender factors to consider, and SPA and pregnancy due to rape. In addition, MHP study participants reported some of the many CITs that may occur during a session with an adult survivor. Of note were the findings from the MHPs regarding the severe levels of abuse that survivors have been exposed to and the need for practitioners to construct a sense of safety while drawing on their inner strengths when the stories and illnesses they are hearing and seeing in the clients become complex and escalate to a serious level.

In addition, evidence in these studies suggests that the impact of a practitioner's gender during a session with an adult survivor needs to be considered carefully and empathically. Finally, the trauma literature emphasises the significance of practitioners and clients working together to establish a healthy therapeutic relationship (Herman, 1992). However, both cohorts in these studies report that a healthy therapeutic relationship with survivors may not be possible without clinically proven guidelines. Therefore, to add weight to the need for a treatment protocol, Volume Two reports on a sample of the research data results administered by MHP study participants to survivors in Theme Two.

KEY THEME TWO
Modalities and Therapies Practised by MHPs

As Chapter Five outlined, survivors present with various social, physical, and mental health challenges and have often disclosed their symptoms to MHPs and mental health professionals. Theme Two highlights

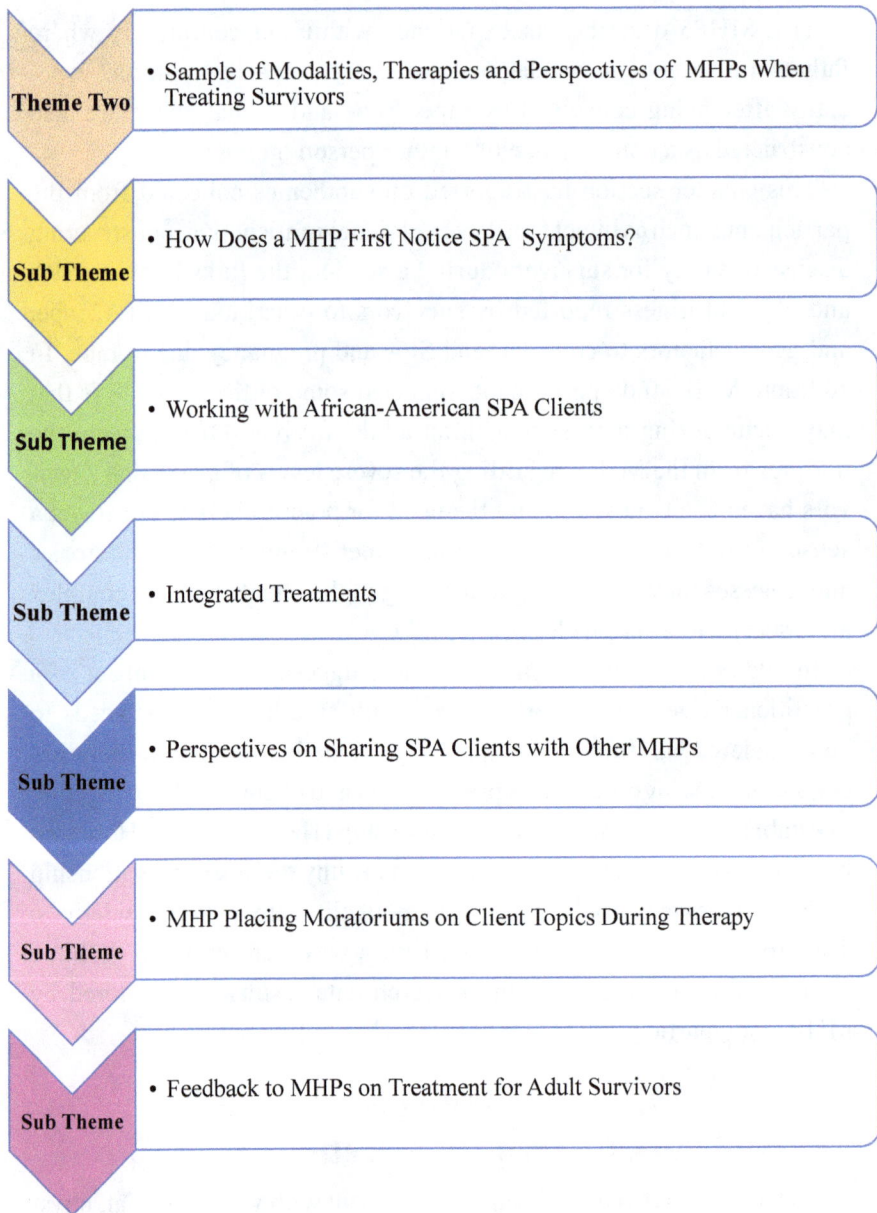

Theme Two
- Sample of Modalities, Therapies and Perspectives of MHPs When Treating Survivors

Sub Theme
- How Does a MHP First Notice SPA Symptoms?

Sub Theme
- Working with African-American SPA Clients

Sub Theme
- Integrated Treatments

Sub Theme
- Perspectives on Sharing SPA Clients with Other MHPs

Sub Theme
- MHP Placing Moratoriums on Client Topics During Therapy

Sub Theme
- Feedback to MHPs on Treatment for Adult Survivors

FIGURE ELEVEN
Main Theme Two and Sub Themes-Modalities, Therapies and Perspectives

the second main theme and subthemes from the interviews with MHP study participants.

Researchers Note to MHPs Regarding Adult Child Survivors of SPA and Filicide

These studies highlight the importance for MHPs to consider whether adult survivors may have been exposed to the CITs discussed in this chapter. MHPs are encouraged to remain vigilant and aware of the potential for adult survivors of SPA to have overheard conversations about filicide or suicide being planned for them or have come close to experiencing such incidents themselves but were intercepted. It is also possible that adult survivors may have experienced such incidents directly but survived the attack and were not killed. Alternatively, it may have happened to a sibling or other family member, such as their biological mother or father. Therefore, it is crucial for MHPs to assess the potential impact of these traumatic experiences on child or adult survivors and to provide appropriate support and interventions to address any resulting psychological distress.

Data were collected regarding the MHP's current methodologies and chosen treatments administered therapeutically to survivors. The practitioners in these studies reported developing their own combination of treatments. In addition, some practitioners reported that they did not know what to recommend while adding that working with survivors can be challenging and working in other areas of the SPA field is 'hideous and high risk' due to their own adverse experiences. For example, difficult areas were described as working within the family court, dealing with targeted APs, being personally and professionally attacked by other PA professionals, and not having a protocol to follow regarding how to work with survivors.

The findings of these studies revealed that MHPs utilise a combination of therapeutic approaches. Additionally, in the data collection process, ten MHPs reported implementing thirty-seven unique therapeutic modalities and therapies when working with survivors. Furthermore, the research findings indicate that while some MHPs chose the same treatment options as their colleagues, other participants utilised an additional thirty-one distinct modalities and therapies. Thus, the data suggests a considerable degree of diversity in the therapeutic approaches used to address the needs of survivors among the practitioners.

Among the thirty-seven treatments and modalities used by the MHP study participants, only one practitioner used the holistic approach of massage combined with counselling, and another used equine therapy with clients. Equine therapy, also known as equine-assisted therapy, is a type of experiential therapy involving horses to help individuals with various mental health or behavioural issues.

Holistic practitioners reported that their choice of methodology and treatment is determined by what they have available and their clients' individual needs and preferences. It is important to note that the list of modalities and therapies administered to survivors by MHPs is only a sample of the study results as the complete results are presented in Volume Three, along with additional information not included in the submitted thesis. Some examples were psychodynamic psychotherapy, existential therapy, emotionally focused therapy, group coaching, mindfulness, play therapy, family systems therapy, exposure therapy and dialectical behaviour therapy, to name a few. Samples of additional information regarding survivors' recommendations for their preferred holistic treatments is presented in Chapter Five, Volume One.

How Does an MHP First Notice SPA?

Within this subtheme, interview results are reported from MHPs who were asked why they believe survivors come to them for therapy and how they begin to work with them. For example, one MHP reflected that the antecedents for survivors to contemplate therapy were many and varied and could include partner relationship and parent difficulties, attachment issues, dysfunctional family patterns, criminal cases related to alienation, and abuse experienced as children. This practitioner also explained the position of moving slowly into a new client relationship. Another practitioner, MHP8, reported that working with SPA clients is highly complex and needs to be handled carefully and over a few sessions until the client gains a deeper understanding of the trauma that they have been through, as explained in the following extract by MHP8;

> Difficulties with relationships that would be the common line. As a family therapist, I ask what the parent's relationship is like, and then the avalanche occurs. And my open questions, because obviously, it's not because it's so traumatic for people, it is not really useful to walk them through it. You know, the old ebb reaction that we used to use with trauma is well and truly dead in the water. The approach now is to stabilise as the first part of the trauma. And so in discussing things, I keep the discussion, you know, kind of up here to begin with (indicated by a raised arm up to her forehead), but usually by the time a first or second session is done, I'm aware of what I'm dealing with. The client won't be though, because they just think it's normal. (MHP8)

In this extract, MHP8 constructs their role as giving the client a gentle entry point to come into therapy. This role is positioned as the practitioner displaying empathy and care for the new client. In MHP8's private practice, their primary client group is adults who have experienced trauma. Consequently, the techniques used can be positioned as raising the importance of being mindful of not pushing a client too quickly during therapy. This technique is constructed as the practitioner making a safe space for the client and assuming the role of 'being careful' while ensuring that they are not acting in a dominating or oppressive way. 'Being careful' safeguards the client while moving them slowly into sessions that may help them to understand that their trauma is not every day. This technique implements knowledge of oneself over their conduct and actions (Foucault, 1988).

A second MHP constructed the intergenerational transmission that follows survivors into a clinical session as an attachment pathology that is "really nasty and severe". This practitioner, 'MHP1', added that "PA is a hidden pathology that fabricates lies and that it is rare for survivors to come into therapy unless they are trying to make meaning of their fragmented lives". Within the following extract, MHP1 reports their perspective on the intrinsic characteristics of survivor experiences and how SPA is closely associated with the secret, hidden levels of lying and normalised abuse that the survivors have suffered as children;

> So, when I'm diagnosing abuse or when I'm encountering it as a psychologist – before the disclosure – you'll see all the signs, you'll see all the themes, but you won't see inside. It's a secret pathology; it's hidden. But you go, wait a minute, I'm seeing stuff here, and then we start to move to help the person disclose. We set the context for the disclosure. We can't go in and look for it because then we distort the evidence. But in the generational transmission, those disperse, and so they move – you can see them in various people, in various processes. And as it moves generations, it gets more and more fragmented. It's a pathology of lies. The child is lying. Everybody's saying, 'everything's normal'. The father's lying to everybody, saying, 'everything's normal'. It's an attachment pathology that is really nasty and really severe. Shame is the other major line in this pathology. Where adults present is when they have come to some degree of awareness, and by that time, they're struggling – and now they're in their older 30s and 40s, and they're trying to figure out what to do and put together a

fragmented life – so they're trying to make meaning of what happened before. (MHP1)

This extract considers the complex issues occurring within the trauma work as the MHP constructs a position of helping to make meaning of the abuse for the survivor. This perspective positions the practitioner as needing to go beyond the apparent presenting trauma symptoms and into the hidden generational constructs that the adult survivor experienced as a child. This stance also allows the practitioner to incorporate the broader historical and social abuse context within a safe environment, allowing the client to safely disclose any shame they may feel due to their child abuse experience. MHP1 constructed their client's complicated feelings stemming from abuse from living within powerful social narratives that can be drawn upon in therapy to situate dysfunctional relationships from the past and present, which give life to a survivor's ideas about fixed identity.

Study data collected from both cohorts have reported that survivors may present with a 'disguised presentation' (Gelinas, 1983) regarding social, physical, and mental health challenges when accessing therapy. Further findings of these studies indicate that several of the survivors sought treatment from general and community mental and physical health professionals to discover that many of them could not help them with SPA (as they did not know about the phenomenon) and unknowingly treated survivors for underlying conditions or symptoms instead of the root cause. Practitioners may reconstruct the 'problem' of SPA abuse as socially constructed when helping the client to challenge any pathological or fixed notions by making space for alternative constructions around the meaning of abuse. These studies' data report that socially constructed abuse is a recurrent pattern in the African-American community. TLE MHP5 offers an example of socially constructed abuse among the African-American community in the USA in the following subtheme.

MHPs Working Within the African-American Population

African-American TLE MHP5 constructs the social patterns of SPA and positions this phenomenon as "being off the charts, yet completely normal when it comes to three to four generations of fatherless homes". For example, in the following extract, TLE MHP5 reports that SPA is generationally taught and culturally adopted by maternal figures spanning decades. Furthermore, TLE MHP5 explains that when clients seek therapy, it is not because they know about SPA. Instead, it is more about the presentation of a hereditary pattern of normalising younger family members not to need fathers, therefore creating a fatherless community requiring SPA patterns to maintain the intergenerational cycle;

They walk into the room, and they have no idea. They say I'm here because I'm an alcoholic. I'm promiscuous. I can't stay married. There's a lot of African-Americans from my country who have really gone through this, and our numbers are off the charts. Many of us grew up in single-parent homes, and other groups culturally don't have this kind of war. This is very new for other cultures. African-Americans are all like, 'your father's nowhere around.' We're desensitised to it. And we've normalised a father not being in the home, even with me expanding to Africa. And we totally accept what mom says. And we go along with that. But yes, I believe it's my grandmother taught me, my grandmother taught my mother or my grandmother taught my mother, my mother taught me. And I've watched three to four generations of women. I've seen how, within the African-American community, there are three to four generations of fatherless homes, and they think it's okay. And they don't know that this is called alienation. They don't know that this is called the measurement. They don't even know this is psychological warfare on their children. They just do what they've been taught to do this intergenerational thing. (TLE MHP5)

In this extract, TLE MHP5 constructs their therapeutic role as being hindered by the expectations from within the sociocultural norms within the African-American communities where she works. According to the Integrated Public Use Microdata Series, "microdata is used to trace race differences in family structure between 1880 and 1980". The high incidence of single parenthood or children living without their parents among African-Americans "is not a recent phenomenon" (Ruggles, 1994, p. 1).

MHP's Perspectives Regarding Treatment for Adult Survivors

The extended literature review for this thesis reported an absence of clear published guidelines for treatments relating to survivors presenting for therapy. As a result, MHPs in these studies tended to adapt their treatment delivery to survivors largely intuitively, using a combination of non-specific and specific therapeutic interventions borrowed from other treatments. This lack of specificity suggests that the centrality of some mechanisms within the action of therapies invariably relies on the probability of change in social communication. The development of an innovative psychosocial treatment model awaits an improved understanding of the biopsychosocial structure that underlies mental health challenges (Fonagy & Luyten, 2019).

A Comparison Between the Field of Mental Health and the Field of Disabilities

The mental health field has fallen behind similar human service fields, such as disabilities. Interestingly, the social model of disabilities has been adopted and dramatically changed since the 1980s to combat how people with a disability were socially constructed negatively. However, in significant contrast to studies on physical illness, the overall frequency of mental illness has not changed within the past 30-40 years (Fonagy & Luyten, 2019). In addition, current treatment therapies can reduce distress in survivors of abuse, but they cannot cure all symptoms due to the lack of established preventative interventions (Fonagy & Luyten, 2019).

A Lack of Formal Training

During the data collection phase of these studies, MHPs offered their perspectives on what they think needs improving regarding treatment options for use with survivors. In addition, the practitioners spoke about a lack of formal training to work with this population and the need for more psychoeducation and research. In the following extract, MHP4, a psychoanalyst and a clinical psychologist with a PhD in neuropsychology, spoke about the dearth of training that is available for MHPs who work with survivors;

> There's no formal training on what you do with adults that I've ever come across. But, the training I'm doing in May identifies the mechanisms by which a child is alienated to become an adult survivor of childhood alienation. And by understanding them, the mechanisms by which a child ends up alienated and takes that into adult life won't stop unless it's interrupted. There's a much greater awareness of how it starts in the mild and moderate phases and much clearer awareness when you're working with adults in a regular psychotherapy room. What you're looking at is the result of severe alienation. In terms of what do you do with an adult who walks in your room? Let's develop a course on here are the skills that you require. Here's the knowledge base, here's what, here's how you should handle it. I don't know anybody who does that. So it's kind of taking information and internalising it and becoming more mindfully aware. And thinking three-dimensionally when somebody arrives in with anxiety and depression, and then the history, you know, you take a history. (MHP4)

In this extract, MHP4 relates how current training is problematised by the fact that awareness has focused on children who have experienced mild and moderate PA but not the severe type in the child or survivors, which is this research's primary focus. MHP4 is a very experienced PA therapist and trainer and has positioned themselves as presenting an educational problem regarding the lack of available courses for MHPs working with survivors of SPA. This problem was highlighted elsewhere within the transcripts by other practitioners.

In the following extract, MHP3 positions themselves as a clinical psychologist unsure of what treatment to recommend and warns about the "dangers and hideousness" of working within the SPA field;

> I'm not even sure what to recommend. It's a hideous situation. It's not a risk-free zone. It's very nasty, as you know. I've talked in the family system sort of approach and tried to explain it with that sort of model, Bowen family systems. I've talked about making connections and how – Bowen's model has self-differentiation in terms of the ability to make contact and still remain a person or an individual. So, I think that's a helpful model. If there was any – and I've tended to be a little bit psychoanalytic and also psychodynamic, but those are the two models I'd probably use. Certainly not CBT! I was running a clinical psych program, but I just don't like CBT. I think it's simplistic, and the whole thing is irrational. How do you bring in rationality into parental alienation? It's not about rationality, it's about something much more dynamic and – probably, attachment theory would be another. I probably talk about it in terms of attachment theory with conflicted or anxious attachment, which tends to be a bit unstable. (MHP3)

In this extract, MHP3 positions themselves as an expert MHP who engage in difficult therapeutic work, often in Family Court, which subsequently constrains them. MHP3 is hindered by not knowing what treatment to recommend and constructs the field of PA and SPA as "hideous and high risk" due to their own experiences. This constraint is additionally significant for MHP3 as many of their clients are distressed, and the treatments MHP3 administers are constructed from a combination of available treatments with specific therapies for other types of trauma. MHP3 also shares that cognitive behaviour therapy (CBT) was administered during a program they were running to treat survivors of trauma but positions themselves as finding this model "simplistic and irrational" and chooses not to use it within a SPA context due to the dynamic and irrational conflict playing out within the phenomenon.

Integrated Treatment

Counselling and Massage

Generally, MHPs apply well-known, common, medically based treatments when working with survivors of abuse; however, one TLE MHP shared that they do not believe that just talking to a person is enough, so, within their practice, they have constructed a different set of professional skills for themselves. As such, they now incorporate counselling and massage. Within this subtheme, the following abstract captures TLE MHP10's construction of an alternative view of their role in addressing SPA trauma by using a "more trusting, hands-on massage approach" in their treatment rooms. This practitioner offers a combination of clinical counselling and massage to access a person's pain within their body to augment healing;

> I never set out to just do massage to make people feel happy, better, and relaxed. All my intention was to allow healing in the person. And wherever the pain in the body, I would move with that. And somehow allow myself to respond to whatever was in a person's beliefs. One comes immediately to mind. I was doing her legs. She just began to cry and say, Oh, my God. It's so painful. And they didn't know what the pain was about. But I knew, because of work that I've done, that they were in pain, obviously, of wounding that they had pushed it down into the legs. I know how her feelings got locked off.

I asked her a few pertinent questions, you know, like, what does it feel like? Is anything coming to you? She was full of tears. And it wasn't just listening and talking and having them try to tell me what was happening for them. We kind of came through the body, and the body can't lie, see, body can't lie. And the body knows if we're willing to listen. (TLE MHP10)

This extract offers an alternative treatment combination for MHPs who work with the impact of traumatic experiences on a client's body by administering a hands-on approach of physical bodywork and talk therapy. As explained in Herman's (1998) model, interventions become one of empowerment and reconnection as the route to recovery (Herman, 2002). With the prevalence of numerous forms of abuse (Boonzaier & de la Rey, 2004) within our communities and the reported impact that abuse can have on clients' lives, TLE MHP10 demonstrates the concept of thinking outside the clinical model when treating clients with trauma. This practitioner constructs an argument that mental health and physical illness may produce symptoms felt as pain within the body and that massage may be offered if the practitioner is confident in their skills and the client feels this may help them heal.

This position is supported by van der Kolk (2014), a psychiatrist who has studied treatments that move away from standard drug and talk therapies and toward an alternative approach that heals the brain, mind, and body. One of these therapies is massage. According to van der Kolk (2014), conventional trauma treatment often overlooks the importance of assisting individuals in safely experiencing their sensations and emotions when they are in a state of fear. Van der Kolk (2014) explains that it is a natural human response to alleviate distress by seeking touch, hugs, and gentle movements. Consequently, he advocates for all his patients to explore various forms of bodywork, such as therapeutic massage, Feldenkrais, or craniosacral therapy, to promote healing and well-being (van der Kolk B, 2014). However, TLE MHP10 has encountered challenges when collaborating with psychiatrists who share the same clients but do not believe in alternative therapies.

Perspectives on Sharing Clients with Other Professionals

Within this subtheme, TLE MHP10 positions their professional work with clients as being problematised by other MHPs and professionals (namely psychiatrists) who place a moratorium on allowing clients to talk about their childhood and then place the clients into mental health units to be heavily medicated when they do not respond to the psychiatrist's treatment;

> One of my PA clients was in such a traumatic state when I met up with them because they were about to put her into a psychiatric hospital and be heavily medicated. I could feel the courage in her that she was willing to stand up and say, it's not where I need to be. So, I trusted her and, and said, Okay, let's find another way, you know, and we can see what's causing the upsets in you and stuff. I really did a lot of work with her body. Just massaging her.

> Another psychiatrist worked with another client of mine. He was giving out medication but not necessarily working with the person. So, he didn't do anything with them. But basically, it's a matter of making sure you have the right tools. Preferably things that they liked when they were a child, like puzzles. But the psychiatrists never attempted to take anything the girl spoke about into consideration. They never, ever helped and then she was so upset, and there was too much time between visits. (TLE MHP10)

From this extract, TLE MHP10 constructs their role as disconnected from their psychiatrist colleagues, whom they perceive as not providing or allowing listening or talk therapy to their mutual clients before placing them in a psychiatric facility. TLE MHP10 also expresses how psychiatrists constrain her work, especially when they do not consider providing inner child work to clients who have been wounded as small children. TLE MHP10 constructs their therapeutic methods amalgamated with massage as giving empowerment, choice and control to clients working with their childhood wounds. "They've got to do it for their own child. I can't do it for the child. They've got to do it. Then I can hold them and support them while they allow the child to come through." (TLE MHP10)

In the following extract, TLE MHP10 establishes a therapeutic approach centred on empowering the client, emphasising the importance of practitioners providing compassion and understanding without judgment or labelling to counteract any potential negative impact from prior psychiatric treatments and shares;

> She was a child of SPA and had been sexually abused, too. And I think that that adds another trauma. She couldn't settle unless we held her and massaged her. Sometimes, it's not all about just headwork and medication. The psychiatrist never took her back. It's also not about the labels. Sometimes, I'm the only safe anchor in the world for these clients. (TLE MHP10)

MHP Perspectives on Placing Moratoriums on Clients' Histories

Within this subtheme, the following extract by MHP7 constructs the workshop boundaries for the treatment practised when working with children of SPA during a week-long court-mandated family reunification program. In contrast to the previous practitioner, who held sessions with their adult client over many months, MHP7 runs workshops for one week with children up to eighteen years old. In addition, this practitioner adopts the position that there should be a moratorium on speaking about the past when working with children of SPA in workshops and also survivors in therapy, and draws from narratives derived from Desmond Tutu and Nelson Mandela to justify their stance;

> There's a moratorium on history. History is filled with irreconcilable perspectives and perceptions. And you can't live there. So, the workshop starts out with that. There's more towards a new family dynamic. And if you know, Desmond Tutu and Mandela can do the amnesty thing, you know, in South Africa, that's what you have to do. You actually set it; you have to let go. And what's important is moving forward and being, you know, in the here and now and appreciating what's happening. So it's, in your experience, it's moving forward. And you have to accept that. That's critical. So, part of the treatment, the education, is to help them understand. There's educational material that really works. It's powerful. They're gonna need to let go, and they need to understand that. (MHP7)

MHP7 constructs a view of boundaries, amnesty, and moratoriums drawn from two famous historical and cultural leaders. These men were compared to Mother Teresa and Pope John Paul 2 (McGowan, 2021). MHP7 clarified their position of implementing a moratorium on children of SPA, focusing on past traumas. They explained that the one-week workshop is more focused on PA education and is not a counselling workshop. MHP7 believes that education on PA is vital and that moving on from the past is critical to the workshops.

In the hope of understanding the practitioners' reference to moratoriums more clearly, the Researcher searched for a link about children not speaking about the past (as per reference to Nelson Mandela). Unfortunately, the only articles related to the moratorium were about Nelson Mandela's announcement to end the death penalty, ending the state of emergency and releasing political prisoners in Africa on February 2, 1990 (Kotze, 2020). In contrast to the views of MHP7, the following example given by TLE MHP10 forms a personal example narrative that a moratorium on speaking about her childhood may not have helped her inner child to heal where her trauma has derived from;

> Some therapists have a moratorium on not talking about your childhood. I know I couldn't have done the healing work I've done without having access to all that happened to me. The damage gets done to the little one, the inner child; that's basically where the trauma comes from. Because, you know, I've not been wanted, that's, you know, like, I can sort of just feel that in every fibre of my being, you know, and it's like, you're little, and you don't know. (TLE MHP10)

The previous extracts by TLE MHP10 and MHP7 highlight the different approaches used by these MHPs when working with survivors of SPA. For example, TLE MHP10 constructs the position based on a personal understanding of what it feels like to be an unwanted child and emphasises the therapeutic value of talking to heal the inner child. TLE MHP10 also asserts that there must be no moratorium for clients to speak about their past abuse, especially those who have experienced CSA. This practitioner draws on psychology and natural remedies such as massage, which historically and currently is used to treat CSA in Indian and Pacific cultures (Galanena, 2019). In contrast, MHP7 believes that imposing a moratorium on discussing past trauma is the best way to work with children within limited time frames while advocating for longer-term therapy for survivors.

These studies note that not having a treatment protocol for survivors could create ethical dilemmas when MHPs disagree, especially when the practitioners are colleagues working with the same patient. These studies also report differences of opinion between MHPs who have lived experience versus those who do not. Once a protocol is designed, these differing opinions must be considered, as previous research reports that ethical dilemmas in medicine are complex and relatively common (Silva et al., 2018).

MHPs and Ethics

Research shows that numerous ethical dilemmas in medicine are related to extraordinary clinical cases almost daily (Silva et al., 2018). In addition, ethical dilemmas are described as typical within a mental health setting due to mental health challenges, causing patients to lack capacity regarding decisions for themselves (Silva et al., 2018). Patients may also depend on MHPs to look after their best interests regarding the law and ethics (Silva et al., 2018). Ethical tensions may also happen because the care of patients with mental health challenges is provided by clinical teams comprising differing staff with differing views, roles, and responsibilities (Silva et al., 2018).

Feedback on Treatment From Survivors, as Reported by MHPs

In the following extract, MHP2 constructs the feedback experiences offered by survivors they have worked with as a dilemma that has been problematic due to clients leaving and never getting in touch again. Conversely, MHP2 reconstructs the narrative of survivors who have provided feedback as a primarily positive experience; however, they worry that they may have "screwed them up" in some way. MHP2 states that they adjust their therapeutic work closely to allow the client to attain a more empowered "end" result. This collaborative method challenges some of the traditional models, for example, the medical model, where the client often plays a more passive part in their treatment when receiving therapeutic intervention from a perceived expert. In contrast, MHP2 takes the position that empowerment for the client must take a leading role;

When I've had feedback, it's always been positive. This is the dilemma – the ones that never talk to you again. You don't know if you've screwed them up or what because they don't talk to you. But the ones that have come back to me, often over the space of years, have said, "If it wasn't for you", etcetera or "I'm always grateful for what you helped me discover". We're always incrementally adjusting how we're working with each other because the end result is the outcome is they're empowered in some way, according to their model of what empowerment actually is. (MHP2)

In this extract, MHP2 discusses the dichotomous and unresolved space that accompanies a lack of feedback from clients who drop out of therapy unexpectedly. The topic can be unsettling and one that MHPs must learn to tolerate when working with survivors of SPA trauma. For example, an article on dropout rates affecting clinicians reports that one in five clients will leave psychotherapy before their treatment is complete (Chamberlin, 2015). Chamberlin (2015) also reports that it can be demoralising for therapists to have clients leave after they have put a lot of time and effort into their treatment, and consequently, they may feel rejected in some ways if a client does not return. This article further reports that practitioners utilising different therapy modalities with SPA clients experience the same dropout rates, even though some psychologists argue that one modality may be superior to another (Chamberlin, 2015).

Conclusion

Theme Two, 'Methodologies and Treatments Practised by MHPs', reported on subthemes collected from the MHP cohort. Subthemes included how MHPs first start to work with survivors presenting for a session, the normalising of fatherlessness within the African-American population, practitioner perspectives on treatment and modalities they administer to SPA clients, sharing clients with other professionals, moratoriums on topics during treatment, ethics, and feedback from clients. Study participants reported some of the many modalities and treatments they may use during a session with an adult survivor.

Finally, the study participants reported practising thirty-one more different modalities and treatments. These figures support the research within the extended literature review in Chapter Three, Volume One, which reported on the dearth of SPA literature regarding treatment protocols.

KEY THEME THREE
Recommendations for Professional Training and Development

part of the study, the ten MHPs were asked which subjects they would recommend to colleagues intending to work professionally with survivors. The recommended modalities and treatments culminated in a collection of subjects that current practising study participants deemed essential, reported upon in Volume Three.

Study participants recommended that potential colleagues undertake a combination of their suggested subjects before working with survivors due to the complexity of the trauma involved. Ongoing clinical supervision for new practitioners in the SPA field was also suggested by 90% of the participants. In addition, professional training and development explicitly supporting practitioners who would like to work with survivors was constructed as lacking in availability by 100% of the MHP participants and some survivors in these studies (Refer to Chapter Five, Volume One).

Recommended Subjects and Topics

The following sample of the final results reports on the recommended specialty subjects and topics that MHP study participants have undertaken to work with survivors. The sample of recommended specialty

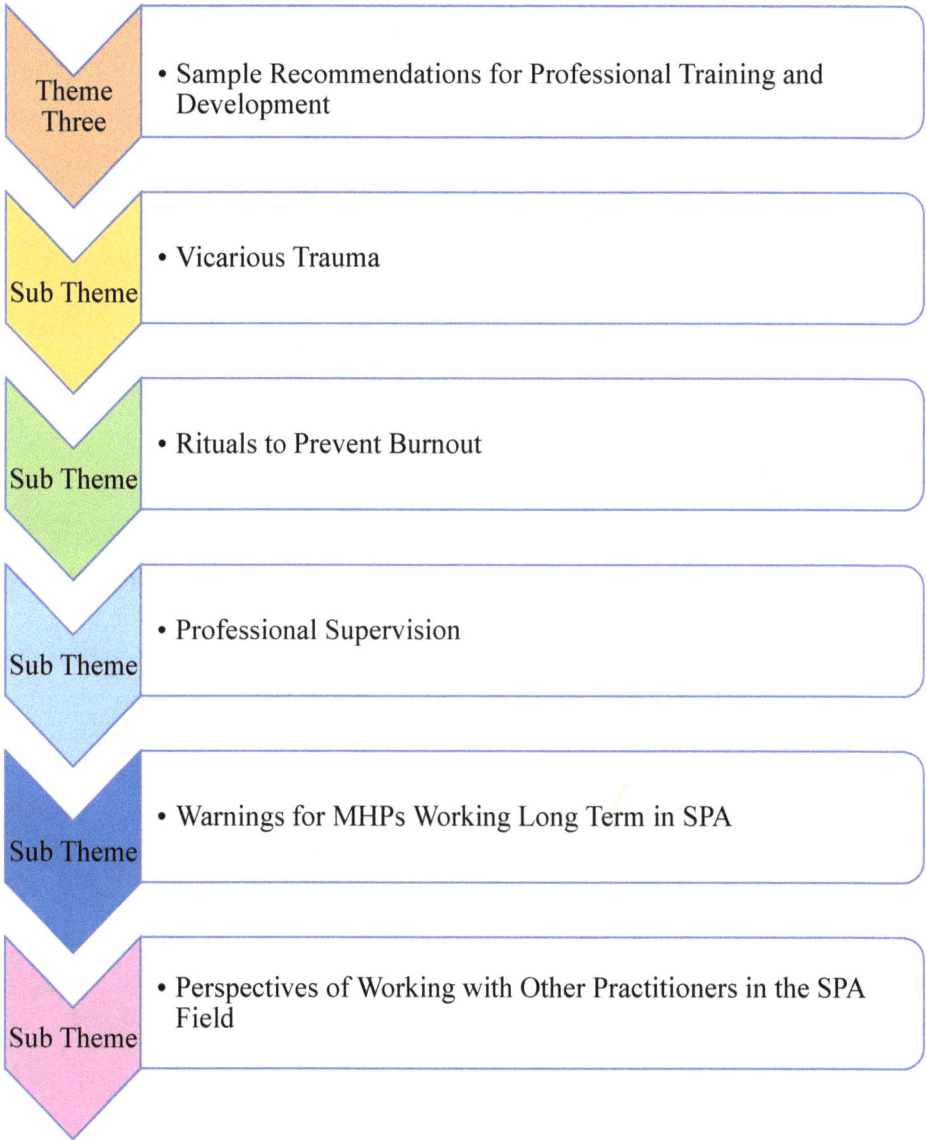

Theme Three
- Sample Recommendations for Professional Training and Development

Sub Theme
- Vicarious Trauma

Sub Theme
- Rituals to Prevent Burnout

Sub Theme
- Professional Supervision

Sub Theme
- Warnings for MHPs Working Long Term in SPA

Sub Theme
- Perspectives of Working with Other Practitioners in the SPA Field

FIGURE TWELVE
Main Theme Three and Sub Themes- Recommendations for Professional Training and Development

subjects to work with adult survivors, as stated by the MHPs, are complex family dynamics, access blocking, boundaries of competence, child abuse, captivity, cognitive distortions, delusional pathology, discourse lenses, false memory syndrome, family therapy training, fear, grief, neuroscience, polyvagal work, relationships, standards of practice for competence and the ideology of family violence to name a few. (Please refer to Volume Three for the full results list.)

Within the seventy-two subjects, only five subjects were repeated. From this data, the other sixty-seven recommended subjects were stated once. This finding is particularly interesting as 100% of the MHPs have worked with survivors, yet most do not have formal training in SPA. An interesting finding emerged among the MHP study participants when each participant recommended different subjects to their counterparts. This means there was no overlap or repetition in the suggested subjects for new practitioners in the SPA field. The lack of overlap or repetition in the recommended subjects suggests a lack of consensus among the participants. This implies that there is no universally agreed-upon set of subjects considered relevant for newcomers in the SPA profession.

Furthermore, different MHPs may prioritise different areas of knowledge and expertise. The wide range of recommended subjects highlights the diverse perspectives among the SPA MHPs. Each participant may have drawn from their own experiences, prior knowledge, or personal beliefs to suggest subjects they deemed important for new practitioners. This diversity reflects the multifaceted nature of CITs in SPA and the variety of approaches and knowledge bases professionals bring.

The diverse recommendations may indicate that the SPA field offers specialisation and niche skills opportunities. New practitioners can consider different subjects based on their desired specialisation, allowing them to discover a unique professional niche within the broader SPA CITs. For example, SPA and abduction, SPA and FDV, SPA and suicidality. However, the lack of consensus on recommended subjects suggests that the SPA areas continuously evolve. New research, emerging practices, and changing client needs may contribute to shifting priorities and perspectives. This highlights the importance of ongoing learning and adaptation for professionals to stay current and responsive to the evolving demands of SPA research and practice.

Additionally, the Researcher argues that a recommended training curriculum and ongoing structured professional development are needed to work with SPA clients. The Researcher also claims that the constraints in MHP training arise from higher education institutions' lack of subject offerings, particularly in specific SPA training, ethics, codes of practice, and clinical work.

Lack of a Code of Practice Standards

For example, MHP1 was particularly troubled about the lack of competent therapists in the SPA field and positioned themselves as coming from an ethically based 'code of practice standards'. This practitioner cited that the existing standard of practice for competence in health care, medicine, and psychiatry does not include standards for working with SPA clients. MHP1 believes that many practitioners are not adhering to current practice standards, let alone specialised standards for SPA and are harming their clients. The following extract is an example of the levels of incompetence and malpractice that MHP1 is concerned about;

> It's attachment, it's complex trauma, it's personality disorders, it's child development, it's family systems, it's self-psychology, and it's the DSM diagnostic system of delusions and thought disorders and child abuse. You need to know what you're doing. And the standard of practice for competence is to know everything there is to know about the pathology and then read journals to stay current. If you're going in for heart surgery, don't you want your heart surgeon to know everything there is to know about heart surgery and be reading the journals to stay current? If your child's getting treated for cancer, don't

you want your child's cancer doctor to know everything there is to know about cancer? Yes, absolutely. You don't want a specialist heart surgeon to look after your sick child if they have brain cancer, yet many MHPs within the field of PA and SPA are not trained to a benchmark standard. That's the standard of practice for competence in health care and medicine, psychiatry and everywhere else except here! And right now, we have zero standards. You're not allowed to be incompetent; that's called malpractice in health care. (MHP1)

In this extract, MHP1 positions themselves as knowing the ethical requirements for other MHPs when working with survivors. MHP1 constructed a narrative of professional concern regarding the lack of standards of practice and competency offered and taught to MHPs working with survivors. MHP1 was the only participant in the study to speak about specific standards of practice that must be developed and followed among PA and SPA professionals working with survivors. Not having the other study participants mention competence in health care or medicine when treating survivors is particularly concerning.

According to a book chapter written by The National Library of Medicine (NLM), there are a set of simple core competencies that all mental health clinicians should adhere to, despite their discipline, to allow the needs of the 21st-century healthcare system to be met (National Library of Medicine, 2003). However, The NLM also states, "The extent to which current health professionals are implementing these competency areas does not meet the health care needs of the American public (National Library of Medicine, 2003, p. 16). These statements validate the narrative that MHP1 is reporting in this research.

The Concept of Harm

The concept of harm is critical when applied to children and survivors. Harm refers to the negative impact of SPA on the mental, emotional, and physical well-being of survivors, their families, and future generations. For example, for child survivors of SPA, the trauma of being caught in the middle of a contentious divorce or experiencing the alienation of one parent can lead to emotional, psychological, and social difficulties. Children may feel conflicted loyalty, guilt, and confusion, leading to long-term negative consequences in their relationships, self-esteem, and mental health.

For survivors, harm may manifest as a range of symptoms, including anxiety, depression, low self-esteem, post-traumatic stress disorder (PTSD), and other mental health challenges. Harm from SPA can also lead to a breakdown in family relationships, including estrangement from one or both parents, siblings, and extended family members. The ongoing conflict and hostility between family members can create a sense of isolation and a lack of support for survivors.

MHPs and Vicarious Trauma

Herman (1992) proposes that support is needed for individuals who work with clients experiencing trauma and recommends, "Just as no survivor can recover alone, no therapist can work with trauma alone" (Herman, 1992, p. 141). The majority of MHPs in these studies explained that their formal study left them ill-equipped and needing to find their own avenues of research in their personal time and at their own expense to understand PA and SPA, combined with connection with other peers to work with such complex levels of trauma.

TLE MHP8 adopted the position of PA not being a clean-cut profession when working with SPA clients and explained, "Okay, so you have no clue what profession you're working in if you think it's clean-cut. If clinicians don't realise what they're looking at is vicarious traumatisation, that's a real worry". Concerningly, 80% of the MHPs in these studies reported that they experienced high levels of vicarious trauma when working with children and survivors of high-conflict divorce, PA and SPA.

Challenges Reported When Working in the SPA Field

According to these studies, 90% of MHPs acknowledge personal challenges when working in the SPA field. The following Table Five lists 83 excerpts from the MHP study participants, highlighting their challenges. These challenges encompass a range of physical and mental health indicators. Furthermore, the table includes general comments, advice, and warnings from various contexts such as group practice, private practice, the public sector, social media, conferences, and the Family Court.

TABLE FIVE
Mental and Physical Health Challenges Reported by MHPs

Challenges
Generalised physical illness
Tachycardia
Feeling nauseated
Feeling violated
Feeling rage
Emotional toll
High stress
Leukaemia
Burnout
PA pract onersleaving the field
Affects to the polyvagal nervous systems
Affects to the autonomic nervous systems
Warnings about working in the SPA field
Being threatened by clients and their families
Being threatened by other PA experts
Being threatened by PA trolls

Needing a bodyguard when Ispeak at conferences
Feeling in danger at work
Threats of being dereg stered due to complaints about reports I've written for the Court
Stress from being cross-examined when appearing in Court as an expert witness
Receiving letters of complaint from the Health Complaints Commissioner
High emotional impact
Vexatious complaints from clients' ex-partners or ex's families
Feeling bruised after some clients and their Court cases
Experiencing accusat ons against you
Feeling unsafe at work
Becomingan excitement junkie
Getting used to the highleve s of trauma the clients have experienced
Becomingdesensit sed to survivor trauma
losing empathy and compassion for clients
Carrying too much trauma in your body from the stories
Watching all the emot ons all the time Becomingtoo drained
Feeling exhausted
Feeling the client's desperat on
Frustrat on from not havine a 2ood treatment for clients
Long processing and debreiefing during personal time after difficult clients
Supporting colleagues such as school principals, lawyers, and Court workers w vicarious SPA trauma
Experiencing a drip feed of stress

Worry all the time
Taking this stuff home to my family
Experiencing disassociated clients too often
Feeling dysregulated
Having panic attacks
Watching children in serious child abuse and feeling helpless
Not being able to function properly with other pat ents after really hard sessions
Reeling from stories of abuse from adult survivors
Dealing with the impact of a shortage of PA professionals in Court
Shortages of custody and access assessors working in Family Court due to the amount of sickness they're experiencing
Huge physical toll
Counselling children and adolescents with terminal illness due to SPA trauma
Resentment about the PA field
Having disgruntled clients find things that you may have done wrong so they can have you deregistered because you can't cover every base all the time
Horrible experiences in Court
Dealing with people at the worst times in their lives
Feeling mangled by clients
Dealing with 'frequent flyer' complainants
Dealing with stressed-out supervisees
Complaints about my lack of intelligence
Losing count of how many complaints I have had aimed at me
Every single complaint sounds like you've run off with somebody and had sex with them. It's over the top!

Having to justify charging higher rates to clients to offset the trauma
If you're in the front line often enough, you can become part of the drama triangle itself
It's just such dangerous work
It's extremely rare for a stranger abduction to be recovered. That's a really hard part of my job. They're usually dead.
When the alienating parent is a member of a cult, that's a double whammy
Maybe 10% of all the PA cases I work with are members of a cult as well
Dealingwith parents with severe personality disorders is extremely stressful
The complexity of family therapy is just that it can be really messy
Ethically, I won't work with anybody who is continuing to be violent towards another
Watching older sons dysregulating and being·violent·to·their·siblings due·to watching their parents fighting
A lot of times I hope to God that the Court practitioner un derstands the parental alienation dynamic in front of them and doesn't become enmeshed with the client. That's my nightmare
Watching someone go from being an advocate to being very dark when they lose their hope. And before you know it, someone's either killed them or they've committed suicide
I'm supporting a judge who's been threatened online. Someone told the judge they would kill him
And the saddest part is when they die, or something happens
And he runs her down, and he kills her as well with the kids sitting in the car. How do I deal with tha t? PA pushed him over the edge

Effectively, some of these adult children were child soldiers. In some cases, the adult children may have been dangerous to their alienating parent, as in trying to kill them, not through any fault of the children, it just is. That's what they were taught. That's what they live with. Somehow, I have to work with that. PA can be A moral
I work with a subset of guys that seem to get off on impregnating women and showing how masculine they are.
So, it's not a risk-free zone, and it's very hard once you become unsafe and are seen to be intrusive in someone's life
How do you work with people who are accusing the targeted parent of sexual abuse when they're not being sexually abusive or domestic violence when they're not being domestically violent?
What used to bug me the most wasthat they were so smug and self-righteous about it, protecting the child when they were clearly damaging the child and ju st couldn't see it
There's no treatment at all. It's a persecutory delusion. You cannot treat it. You cannot work with it. You cannot challenge it.

In the following extract, MHPs construct the position that when they engage in trauma work with survivors of SPA, they can be subject to vicarious trauma that may manifest in physical health challenges. The study participants caution that practitioners must be aware of and actively try to prevent vicarious trauma from occurring when engaging in therapeutic work. For example, MHP4 constructs the day and time according to when demanding clients are due to attend a session to reduce their trauma impact, including the manifestation of difficult physical symptoms within themselves;

> I have developed symptoms of tachycardia before going into
> a room. I regularly have digestive issues before and after
> sessions, nausea, and feeling violated. Rage just wanting to

impale them on something for their myopic approach to their children. I have to be very careful when I say see them in my clinical week and what time of day I see them. I will often see them the last piece of the day because if I were to see them in the middle of the day, I would not be able to function with my other patients. It gives me my drive home to process what happened. Luckily, there are a group of people that I found that are just trained, and we can call each other up and process with someone else who knows how difficult the work is and kind of bounce back. And so, there's a huge physical toll. (MHP4)

Reports of Cancer Among MHPs

These research findings also revealed that one MHP study participant reported that five MH professionals at their place of work have cancer, which they believe relates to working in the PA field, and another one (equalling six) was experiencing aggressive leukaemia. Additionally, one of their adolescent clients was diagnosed with cancer. Subsequently, in the last three weeks, an individual report received via email to the Researcher about another PA researcher being diagnosed with cancer came through. This email revealed that the researcher referred to in the email has developed an aggressive form of breast cancer.

Occupational Cancer

The data from these studies highlight a concerning pattern of potential cancer links among survivors and MHPs within their immediate collegial social circle. Importantly, even though the MHP who reported the coworkers with cancer believed it was due to PA, this hypothesis needs further investigation. However, the reported data is still significant because it has not been documented in previous studies to the Researcher's knowledge.

Further investigation and attention to these connections are warranted to better understand the underlying factors and potential vicarious trauma implications for the health and well-being of those affected by SPA. For example, if six MHPs in the same building all have cancer or leukaemia, several factors could be at play. Another reason for the high incidence of cancer in the MHPs' workplace could be 'occupational cancer'. Occupational cancer is the development of cancer primarily or partially attributed to exposure to carcinogens in the workplace (Canadian Center for Occupational Health and Safety, 2023).

Scientific studies indicate that the extent of cancer cases related to occupational hazards differs depending on the specific type of cancer (Canadian Center for Occupational Health and Safety, 2023). The prevalent forms of occupational cancer include lung, bladder, and mesothelioma (Canadian Center for Occupational Health and Safety, 2023). It is important to note that identifying specific causes would require a thorough investigation and analysis by experts in occupational health and environmental factors.

Subsequently, the Researcher proposes that potential factors that could be considered in such a scenario include: Environmental factors: The building or its surroundings might be exposed to specific environmental hazards or toxins, such as asbestos, radon, mould, or chemicals, which could contribute to the development of cancer or leukaemia (Wurtz et al., 2020). Occupational hazards: MHPs may be exposed to occupational hazards in their work environment, such as radiation (e.g., X-rays in diagnostic imaging), chemotherapy drugs, or other hazardous substances used in treatment or research settings (American Cancer Society, 2023).

Additionally, shared risk factors: The MHPs may share common risk factors for cancer or leukaemia, such as certain genetic predispositions, lifestyle factors (e.g., smoking, excessive alcohol consumption), or personal medical history (Larsson et al., 2020). Also, a chance occurrence or cluster: A cancer cluster is described by the US Centers for

Disease Control and Prevention (CDC) and the National Cancer Institute (NCI) as an occurrence where the number of cancer cases surpasses what is typically anticipated, affecting a specific group of individuals residing in a well-defined geographic region during a particular time-frame (American Cancer Society, 2023). It is essential to consider that the clustering of cancer or leukaemia cases among the MHPs may be coincidental, as cancer can occur randomly in any population (American Cancer Society, 2023).

Furthermore, stress and burnout may be the cause: High levels of chronic stress, emotional strain, and burnout among MHPs could impact their immune system and overall health, potentially increasing the risk of cancer (Jaber, 2021). Also, occupational or lifestyle exposures may be involved. For example, assessing if the practitioners have common exposures outside their workplace, such as hobbies, second jobs, or personal habits, that could contribute to their increased risk is crucial. In any case, determining the exact factors contributing to the presence of cancer or leukaemia among the MHPs would require a thorough investigation by relevant authorities, including environmental health experts and occupational health specialists, who can conduct comprehensive assessments and studies to identify potential occupational or environmental hazards.

The Manifestation of Physical Illness Among Practitioners

In the following extract, MHP4 discusses the emergence of physical symptoms within a clinical psychologist's human social experience. MHP4 has positioned physical health indicators as unavoidable for the practitioner during therapy and explains that symptoms must be openly and honestly addressed. This practitioner further emphasises the need to construct a level of outside support from neutral, non-judgemental professionals in the SPA field to offset the impact of vicarious trauma. These experiences create the position of the clinical psychologist needing to consider any incidents they encounter and carry within themselves, which are deemed as shaping and constructing the practitioner. MHP4 also spoke about serious, long-term physical illness among their peers;

> There was a group of social workers, predominantly some psychologists, who had a group practice, and they worked in the realm of high-conflict divorces, so many of them were custody and access assessors. There may be six professionals in that building. Every single one of them had cancer. And it wasn't until I was educating how the damage to children occurs through the hypothalamus pituitary adrenal axis in the body and made reference to the physical illnesses that one of them shared that they had been unwell and ended up diagnosed with a very rare leukaemia, which is public knowledge, or I wouldn't be sharing this with you. (MHP4)

The previous extract is an intriguing finding of the study. The fact that the MHPs believe that they are becoming unwell due to working in the field of SPA is an ironic point that builds on data reported earlier in this chapter, where the MHPs were showing concern about SPA clients and the illnesses they presented within a session. The research data now indicates that both the survivors of SPA and the MHPs may be experiencing illnesses due to exposure to SPA, no matter what type of SPA work they are undertaking or where. For example, the following subtheme is constructed from the high impact on practitioners and their colleagues who work within the Court system on cases involving SPA.

Vicarious Trauma from Working in Court

In the following extract, MHP3 reconstructs the experiences of ongoing nastiness they have experienced in family court;

> I was a court expert for probably 15 years, and that was up until about 2008 – 2009. And I remember complaining – I

used to go with the Judges and other court professionals to the Christmas parties, and I just used to feel so bruised, year after year. Then I got this case, which was truly nasty, and I mean it was so nasty that the lawyers, magistrate, etc., had a bit of a Christmas party after the case resolved to just console one another. I'm talking about both sides, child rep. Everybody got together and had drinks just to get over the trauma of these unbelievably ugly people. Now, this person actually managed to get something that I got cautioned on, so it was probably the worst result I had with the complaints commissioner; he not only put in a complaint, but he got something to stick, which is usually pretty difficult. So, it's not a risk-free zone, and it's very hard once you become unsafe. I had a weekly peer supervision group, which we used to meet for an hour, and I would have extra supervision if I felt I needed it. So, I stopped for five or eight years until I went back to it after I ran a clin psych program and then as a professor. (MHP3)

This practitioner positions Court SPA work as an area that needs ongoing peer and professional support. MHP3 positions themselves as needing to self-surveil regarding the impact of high-conflict divorce on them professionally and personally. The extract is constructed as evoking 'vicarious trauma' in both the MHP and the teams of professionals working in the Family Court system of Australia. This position protects oneself concerning therapeutic discourses of impending vicarious trauma (Adams & Riggs, 2008) caused by hearing high-conflict divorce and SPA accounts within the court systems. This self-preservation may be considered a technology of oneself (Foucault, 1988). Protecting oneself requires MHPs to continuously monitor their feelings and thoughts while intrinsically exploring their intrinsic world to attain the industry-recommended status of 'the self-aware practitioner' to work against any impact on therapeutic conduct (Herman, 2002).

Rituals to Prevent Burnout

Within this sub-theme, the importance of MHPs engaging in rituals to prevent vicarious trauma and burnout was an unexpected finding. When the Researcher searched for peer-reviewed articles on therapist rituals, none were discovered. Consequently, a 'white article' about therapists who work from home and their rituals to prevent burnout was drawn upon. MHPs who were interviewed shared examples such as; they walk into their kitchen and reheat the kettle to reset; they wash their face with warm water; they may do a quick workout; or taking a break from online work while finding a quiet place to breathe (Nesvig, 2022). In addition, MHP8 described the ritual they go through before and during a client session to reduce any vicarious trauma that may occur;

> When it comes to rituals, this is one of the things I do 15 minutes before a session. I don't look at SMSs, voicemails, emails, none of that because what they can do is take me into that space, and I need to be in this space with my client. I will have done that the day before at the latest. I have a lot of clients who dysregulate, dissociate all of that kind of stuff. I have strategies. I have learned how to sit really still. Because when somebody is dissociated, if you move, it can really disrupt the process. If there's something that's particularly awful that I'm hearing about, I have a vacuum cleaner. That's my little vacuum cleaner there. So, I'll rub my finger and thumb together, and we'll be out of view of the client. That way, I can suction out that stuff. It doesn't hit me, and I don't ever sit front on to a client. I always sit slightly angle to protect my polyvagal system as much as possible. (MHP8)

Support from Socially Constructed Groups to Prevent Vicarious Trauma

A systematic review published in Poland on burnout and well-being of psychotherapists concluded that burnout and well-being among this population are related to sociodemographic structures such as intrapersonal and work-related activities (Van Hoy & Rzeszutek, 2022). In the following extract, MHP4 positions themselves as accessing support from socially constructed groups to prevent vicarious trauma. MHP4 also refers appreciatively to their training at university as a psychoanalyst. Finally, this participant refers to the adopted university construct of therapist preparation training, which included psychoanalysis of themselves from their clinical supervisor as part of the course over the years;

> You may know that as part of the training to become a psychoanalyst, one needs to be in psychoanalysis to deal with one's own issues so as not to pass them on and that having had a successful psychoanalysis. Being on somebody's couch four times a week, for years, working through, really strengthens the weave in, in the character of me or any other analyst in training. That helps. It helps that I, I have a love of singing and belong to a rock choir and sing in, you know, for eight-part harmony with 150 people. I love it, and having really good friends and really solid family relationships, that really helps. (MHP4)

Clinical Supervision

In this sub-theme, MHP participants constructed the value of supervision and support from their peers and clinical supervisors as integral and vital for their work. Many of the MHPs in these studies emphasised the merit of peer debriefing and clinical supervision with practitioners who thoroughly understood the phenomena of SPA and its exhausting nature.

Clinical Supervisors Leaving Due to Stories About SPA From Supervisees

The following practitioner reported that their clinical supervisor (whom they needed to teach about SPA during supervision) experienced vicarious trauma from listening to stories from the supervisees' work with their SPA clients and had to leave the sessions. MHP2 shared;

> I actually believe I was in danger of burnout if I didn't do something different. It's draining work. It's been exhausting work spread over several years. I have regular peer supervision debriefing within a core group of PA specialists in Australia to combat burnout. Historically, my clinical supervisor didn't know anything about PA, so I had to teach them. I had pretty good professional supervision until I burnt out my clinical supervisor. So, they actually got vicarious trauma from my PA work, so I had to find another one! (MHP2)

Within the previous extract, the MHP positions themselves at a disadvantage by needing to teach their clinical supervisor about parental alienation to get adequate supervision. Unfortunately, the supervisor became vicariously traumatised from listening to this practitioner's case presentations about SPA and consequently stopped supervision, further disadvantaging the supervisee. Supervisees teaching clinical supervisors about SPA is another interesting and ironic finding because the survivors in the research also mentioned needing to teach the practitioners that they were engaging in therapy about PA and SPA. This finding supports the literature review of these studies (See Chapter Three) that concluded that there is a dearth of research, professional training and psychoeducation in the community being offered and administered within the SPA field.

Warnings for MHPs Working Long Term in the SPA Field

In the following sub-theme, MHP3 constructs the unsafe aspect of report writing, being an expert witness within the Family Court system of Australia and knowing when to leave. Safety is constructed as the ability to leave this system (as they are about to retire) if they get complaints against them from disgruntled PA clients. Therefore, MHP3 needs to pay close attention to the protection of their professional career to make working in the Family Court system safe. In doing so, they offer several insights and personal considerations regarding their career within the extract below.

MHP3, an expert witness and clinical psychologist who has worked for 30 years in The Australian Family Court, warned other practitioners about "getting out of doing work with families in the long term". MHP3 also warned that both vicarious trauma and the professional repercussions of deregistration were due to the dangerous nature of complaints against practitioners. Furthermore, MHP3 explained the dangerous position that he had found himself in as an experienced clinician;

> You've got to get out of family work. I got out of family law for ten years after I had a very bruising experience with a nasty client, and so I took a break, but I've gone back to it in the last two or three years because I believe that there's an advantage to having experienced clinicians who are good at assessment, actually do this work. It's so dangerous because you can get complaints from your registration authority. You can be deregistered for it because they can find things that you've done wrong, and you can't cover every base. So, I figure it's best for me to do it because I don't care if they deregister me because I'm retiring soon anyway. (MHP3)

TLE MHP9 shared the same warning sentiments as MHP3 regarding discussions of vicarious trauma. TLE MHP9 also offered advice regarding the need for MHPs to develop a plan to leave the PA and SPA field due to bullying by parents and other PA professionals. "At some point, you say, fucking excuse my French, sick of dealing with dysfunctional parents and being professionally attacked by PA professionals. I'm glad you're doing this research, but you need to keep developing 'an out' as well." (MHP9)

Perspectives of Working with Other Practitioners in the SPA Field

Accounts of Bullying Among PA Professionals

Within the interviews analysed, MHPs narrated their diverse experiences of bullying aimed at them within the culture of PA and SPA. These accounts included psychological abuse, maintaining silence about PA work to protect their reputations, plagiarism, and professional attacks from other MHPs within the SPA field. A study into workplace bullying in the health field reported that bullying among professionals is a complex yet common phenomenon among healthcare organisations (Zachariadou et al., 2018). In addition, these studies report show that work colleagues play a critical role in identifying being bullied, as well as with the possible causes of bullying, and are central to generating meanings and labels for workplace bullying (Lewis, 2003, p. 65).

Further Removal of Identifiers to Protect MHP Study Participants

Please note that the following extracts have had the MHP's I.D. numbers removed, and they have been deidentified to a greater degree due to the sensitivity of the content. Removing the identifiers adds an extra layer of confidentiality for the practitioners due to the small pool of experts in the PA field, who often know each other. Removing identifiers has also been performed due to threats of violence aimed at some of the MHP study participants from other PA colleagues. For example, one practitioner attends conferences as a speaker with a bodyguard due to threats to their life. Within these predominantly negative experiences, graphic descriptions of the fighting that takes place among some of the expert MHPs were reported as follows;

> And they told me not to tell anybody when I started in the field. It's just so disgustingly embarrassing that the clinicians and researchers are arguing like this. It makes me puke. That's why I really like (removed for confidentiality). I don't agree with everything he says, but he's willing to look at different areas, and he gets attacked by these people. And it's ridiculous, and he's just really about research, you know? Yeah. Interesting guy, and they're just awful, and it's, what has to happen is, first of all, the field has to stop the parallel process. You know, like, I'm afraid to speak at PA conferences. I've been invited many times to go to the PA meetings and to present. I don't want to go because I don't want to be attacked. There's a big war started. A massive war. I've never seen anything like it. They're just taking each other down. (ID withheld for confidentiality)

Manifestations of the Fighting Among PA Professionals

Another MHP openly shared their concern about the fighting that has manifested between the expert PA professionals and shared how traumatic and disturbing it is for the MHPs and survivors who are watching these behaviours;

> I'm very concerned about all the fighting in the PA arena. It's the ones with the newest knowledge, the newest papers, and the longest University tenure. The clients are not being helped when the academics are fighting with each other. They really need to stop. If they all came together, the research would

improve, and parental alienation would be a lot further along than it is. It's deplorable behaviour, really, and the topmost famous researchers are some of the worst. I am trying to work without getting entangled by it. What the top academics and researchers are doing is disturbing for the practitioners watching them. They are supposed to be mentoring us, but they're more interested in their egos and the money they make from the trauma. If they had trauma themselves, they would be stronger advocates. The survivors are angry with them, too. They monopolise the conferences and big-note themselves at every opportunity. They are acting like dinosaurs. Things need to change dramatically. They need to use more emotional intelligence and kindness. (ID withheld for confidentiality)

The deidentified MHP in this extract constructs encountering a 'deplorable behaviour' from another PA professional described as "disturbing and hard to watch". They identify this experience as being in an unwanted and frustrating position while expecting more from the experts who are supposed to be mentoring less experienced practitioners and survivors. This practitioner reported that "experts working in the field of PA at an international level might need to consider who is watching their behaviours and how it affects those who look up to them". (ID withheld for confidentiality)

Plagiarism Among the PA Professionals

Plagiarism among the professionals within PA has also been reported in these studies. For example, one MHP spoke about having their work stolen from a PA expert, who was a developmental researcher, not an MHP and denied having done so. This MHP explained, "I stopped working with them when they took my whole protocol for a project ahead of having the entire thing published, and then when I went to them about it, they were like, oh no, this is mine". (ID withheld for confidentiality)

In the following extracts, two different study participants described the levels of bullying and violence that have been aimed at them by PA members whom they described as experts in the PA field who are trying to solve PA;

Extract 1 "It's just the same domestic violence clients are exposed to. It's just PA experts now doing it. And they can be violent towards each other, and then they're like, oh, no, we're solving PA. And I'm like, just stop it. Like, cut it out. You just don't understand what your behaviour is actually doing. We can't watch it!" (ID withheld for confidentiality)

Extract 2 "Both sides of the fence are not nice. The PA people and the non-PA people are a mess. Yeah, thing is, a big war is about to start, and I'm just staying right out of it because I'm an adult child of severe PA myself. And to me, it's like having mum and dad fighting again and having to pick a side, and I'm like, not doing it. Some of the (withheld PA) people had a go at me, and it's just, it's unfair. And I'm like, screw you guys. I've had a very big name (name withheld) go after me. (Name withheld) also had a go at me in a very nasty way. And it's not okay. If anybody has a 100% cure for anything, let me know. Yeah. I'll be glad. That's all I'm gonna say." (ID withheld for confidentiality)

The previous extracts have shared the themes of violence, bullying, and a lack of non-violent communication (Rosenberg, 2015) and mentorship as experienced by different MHPs, aimed at them by experts in the SPA field. Despite practitioners coming from different countries, they all shared similar experiences, perspectives, and comments about being targeted and bullied. As a result, their collective insights provided a unified global perspective, mirroring the findings of their counterparts in the study.

Chapter Summary

In conclusion, this chapter explored the experiences and perspectives of MHPs who work with adult survivors of SPA. The findings provided valuable insights into various aspects of the MHPs' qualifications, practice areas, backgrounds, and motivations for working in the field of child psychological abuse combined with SPA. One key theme that emerged was the challenging dynamics involved when parents of survivors stay together, separate, or divorce, leading to potential risks of familicide and homicide. The chapter also highlighted cases of abduction and threats of harm, emphasising the grave consequences that the CITs from SPA abuse can have on survivors' lives. Additionally, the relationship between SPA, physical illness among survivors, and the CITs of SPA with issues such as rape and gender were explored, shedding light on the far-reaching impact of SPA on survivors' well-being.

Another key theme focused on the modalities and therapies employed by MHPs in their work with survivors. The chapter discussed how MHPs first notice signs of SPA, particularly within the African-American population, and highlighted the perspectives of MHPs regarding treatment for survivors. The comparison between the fields of mental health and disabilities revealed insights into the need for advancement in the area of PA and SPA to catch up to the disabilities field, formal training and integrated treatment approaches. Furthermore, MHPs shared their experiences collaborating with other professionals, placing moratoriums on clients' histories, and ethical considerations within the SPA field.

The third key theme revolved around recommendations for professional training and development for MHPs working with SPA survivors. The chapter highlighted a sample of suggested subjects and topics that MHPs recommended should be included in training programs and the need for a code of practice standards. Please refer to Volume Three for the complete list of results.

The concept of harm and the impact of vicarious trauma on MHPs were also explored, along with the challenges faced by practitioners in the SPA field. Rituals to prevent burnout, support from social groups, and the importance of clinical supervision were discussed as essential elements in supporting MHPs' well-being and preventing vicarious trauma.

Throughout the chapter, accounts of bullying, plagiarism, and conflicts among professionals in the field of PA and SPA were presented, underscoring the complexities and challenges that can arise within the professional community. Theme Three reported on subjects and topics proposed by MHPs for other professionals interested in working with survivors. Sub-themes raised by this cohort investigated vicarious trauma, challenges faced, rituals to prevent burnout, clinical supervision, warnings to practitioners working long-term in the SPA profession, and perspectives of working with other practitioners. Following on, Chapter Seven provides a summary, evaluation, and implications of the key topics presented in Chapter Five (Adult Survivors' Perspectives, Volume One).

Chapter Seven Conclusion

Significant clinical themes emerged and identified potential novel diagnostic indicators. These findings offer crucial clinical implications, empowering MHPs to better understand and monitor the well-being of SPA survivors within a clinical context. The Researcher recommends further research on the 'specific phobia-severe parental alienation, and abduction anxiety variant' (Price-Tobler, 2023), along with information and links regarding SPA and FDIOA, and FDIOA and malingering by proxy and also shared delusional disorder.

These findings recommend that MHPs and medical professionals consider all potential CITs when working with this complex client group, as it further substantiates the strong association between SPA and trauma as adults. The CITs also serve as a reminder of the extensive toll that SPA can take on individuals' overall well-being. Recognising and addressing physical and mental health issues is essential to provide comprehensive support for survivors through their treating professionals.

✧

Chapter Eight
Study Two - Discussion and Conclusion - Mental Health Practitioners

These studies report that MHP study participants demonstrated a high level of competence and expertise in their chosen areas of mental health while also pursuing a special interest and focus on survivors of SPA. The study also reports on the identified barriers to treatment, including stigma, lack of community awareness, and inadequate funding for SPA mental health services. MHPs emphasise the importance of creating a safe and supportive therapeutic environment for SPA clients to facilitate healing and recovery. The MHPs also reported that clinical supervision is crucial to support their professional development, promote best practices, and prevent burnout.

These studies recommend that a gold standard for competence, training, and ongoing professional development be determined. Creating a gold standard will assist MHPs in understanding the degree, acuity, complexity, and severity of survivors' developmental and ongoing acute trauma, improving their competence and confidence in working with SPA clients. In addition, the lack of SPA-specific training and education in mental health programs highlights the need for curriculum reform.

Furthermore, these studies revealed that some MHPs treat SPA clients without following best practice guidelines, underscoring the need to develop ethical standards. Finally, these studies emphasised the broader social and political implications of SPA, including the impact of SPA trauma on physical health and the need for culturally sensitive and ethical approaches to address SPA trauma in different communities.

Data Collection Themes

The data collected from the MHP study participants provided valuable insights into their levels of professional training, reasons for entering the field, the challenging dimensions they encounter, and the number of SPA cases they have worked with. The research also captured the MHPs' perspectives on CITs, ethical considerations and their experiences with colleagues in the SPA field. Another consideration reported by the MHP study participants includes the need for client-centred therapy, the importance of understanding and addressing the dynamics of PA, SPA and SPAA, the impact of trauma, and the need for building a therapeutic alliance with survivors.

The data collected from the MHP participants in these studies revealed a significant variation in the NUMBER of SPA cases they have worked with. For example, while some participants reported having worked with only a few adult survivor cases, others reported having worked with hundreds. From a mentoring point of view, the more experienced MHPs highlighted the need for specialised training to equip current, less experienced, and future MHPs with the necessary skills and knowledge to identify and treat SPA-related issues effectively.

Complex Intersecting Traumas

The findings of these studies highlight that some MHPs enter the field of SPA due to their intrigue and desire to make sense of the chaos they encounter while working with this complex client group. However, results reported from some of the more experienced MHPs explain that their lack of specific SPA training often presents a challenge regarding recognising symptoms and knowing how to treat them. In addition, the study participants noted that working with survivors can be challenging due to the CITs and underlying symptoms often being overlooked by other MHPs before they present to them for treatment.

This challenge is compounded by the fact that survivors who present may not return due to the MHP not noticing their CIT symptoms. Consequently, survivors may only be treated for symptoms like addiction, sustaining relationships, or physical or mental health challenges. This lack of training makes it difficult for MHPs to gain the necessary knowledge, skills and experience to work effectively with this client group. In addition, the absence of treatment options to use with survivors was also reported as a challenge by MHPs. Furthermore, the MHPs in these studies reported that they were frustrated that many of their colleagues lacked the knowledge and skills to effectively identify and treat underlying SPA issues.

Practitioners reported a kaleidoscope of CITs that survivors spoke about during therapy, such as intact families experiencing physical illness, rape, gender, SPA and CSA, SPA and SPAA and pregnancy due to rape. Of particular concern to the MHPs were the severe levels of abuse experienced by survivors, including threats of familicide and homicide and physical illness due to SPA trauma (Refer to Chapter Five for the extended list provided by the adult survivor study participants).

These studies report that MHPs must consider and explore the CITs the client reveals to work with survivors effectively. The added layers of CITs compound the trauma for survivors, and to help the client heal, these must be watched for and addressed when the client is open and ready. These studies recommend that MHPs and other community professionals familiarise themselves with the myriad of potential CITs that a client may have been subjected to. Familiarising oneself with potential CITs and listening carefully for additional CITs that may not have been captured in the research is recommended.

Lack of Recognition

The lack of training and awareness among MHPs working with survivors is a critical issue that needs to be addressed. It is alarming that some MHPs do not recognise SPA symptoms or investigate if their clients are SPA trauma survivors. This lack of recognition raises questions about the ethical responsibility of MHPs and the potential harm caused by their lack of training to work with this population. Training for MHPs must also focus on the unique needs and experiences of survivors of SPA. This may include training on trauma-informed care, cultural sensitivity, and specific therapeutic approaches until a protocol is developed. These studies recognise that this space is challenging for MHPs to work with and is understanding of their plight. In the immediate future, practitioners must also be trained to recognise the signs of SPA and SPAA and work with survivors to break the cycle of abuse and prevent the intergenerational transmission of trauma.

Professional and Ethical Repercussions

The absence of clear guidelines for treatments and the lack of formal training for SPA and SPAA are major challenges that need to be addressed by the mental health field. It is worth noting that while the Researcher initially omitted the topic of standards of practice for MHPs, it is possible that they were aware of it but chose not to mention it. However, it was later added in response to the emphasis placed by one MHP, highlighting its significance.

This addition sheds light on the absence of clear treatment guidelines and formal training for addressing SPA, presenting significant challenges in the mental health field. These challenges extend beyond individual practitioners to encompass broader professional and ethical ramifications. Specifically, the studies reveal that only one out of ten practitioners in the study mentioned the importance of standards of practice, raising questions about their knowledge of and adherence to professional standards.

Additionally, this lack of attention leaves MHPs ill-prepared to provide effective and ethical treatment to SPA clients, potentially resulting in inadvertent harm to clients and practitioners themselves. Moreover, the absence of specific training and standards of practice raises concerns about the potential detrimental impact on the mental well-being of MHPs, including increased stress, burnout, ethical dilemmas, and risk of secondary trauma. Further investigation into MHPs' awareness and understanding of practice standards is warranted to address these gaps and ensure the delivery of quality care.

Differing Opinions Among MHPs

These studies also highlight the differing opinions among MHPs when working with survivors. The topic of moratoriums was contested in the research. For example, one practitioner, MHP7, believes that a moratorium on discussing past traumas is necessary when working with survivors. However, TLE MHP10 advocates open dialogue on past experiences to facilitate healing. Ethical dilemmas may arise when practitioners disagree, underscoring the need for clear guidelines. MHPs must recognise the potential ethical dilemmas that can arise when disagreements occur and the adverse effects this can have on survivors seeking help. By working together, practitioners can provide consistent and effective care to survivors, ultimately preventing further intergenerational transmission while promoting healing and well-being.

Unfortunately, the research data captured that many survivors of SPA face significant barriers to accessing treatment and support, such as being silenced, a lack of recognition of their trauma, feeling suicidal, or being sent home without receiving adequate care. Therefore, emergency departments, mental health units and other healthcare providers must receive training on SPA and how to provide appropriate care and support to survivors. This includes psychoeducation and training to recognise the signs of SPA and SPAA, providing trauma-informed care, supporting survivors in breaking the cycle of abuse and when where to refer to a different professional (they have investigated as a respectable referral) if they are not trained to help further. These steps are critical because injustice and violence increase in silence. Addressing and stopping the violence associated with SPA and SPAA requires a multifaceted societal approach involving education programs, associations, practitioners, and other community professionals. By raising awareness, providing training and support, and taking action to support survivors, the cycle of abuse and prevention of intergenerational transmission of trauma can be slowed down.

Constructing a Sense of Safety

Data from the study reports that MHPs need to construct a sense of safety for their clients and themselves. A sense of safety is essential for SPA clients, but even more so when working with SPAA survivors who have been abducted or had threats of being killed by a parent, a family member, or a stranger. The MHP study participants suggested that other practitioners must draw on their inner strengths when the stories of SPA trauma and illnesses they are hearing and seeing in the clients become complex and escalate to a severe level. MHPs may also need to construct a sense of safety for themselves concerning the prevention of vicarious trauma in the field of PA and SPA. For example, MHP (ID withheld for confidentiality) also shared that working with clients involved with abduction, homicide detectives, and forensic police attracts people who attack them and make Board complaints against them, not allowing them to feel safe when they work. (Refer to Chapter Six for vicarious trauma results).

Physical Illness Presentations in SPA Clients and MHPs

The MHP study participants reported that physical illness is a significant consequence of SPA trauma for survivors and always needs to be considered when working with SPA clients. This research reported on the high levels of physical illness and ongoing ailments that survivors live with due to childhood trauma. It recommended that partnering with the client's medical team would be advantageous.

Physical and psychological illness among the MHPs was also a concerning factor reported in the results. MHP study participants reported that they and their colleagues become ill due to the high levels of vicarious trauma they are exposed to when working in the SPA field. This data includes MHPs working with children and survivors and alienated TPs. Illnesses listed were tachycardia, panic attacks, leukaemia, and six instances of cancer in colleagues specialising in PA and SPA, to name a few. (Refer to Chapter Six, 'Mental and Physical Health Challenges Reported by MHPs') for an extensive list.

Vicarious Trauma on MHPs

The data collected from MHPs working with survivors highlights the challenges practitioners face when working with such complex cases. The majority of MHPs in the study reported feeling ill-equipped to handle cases of SPA, highlighting a critical gap in the professional training of practitioners in this field. This lack of training and a code of practice leaves MHPs vulnerable to vicarious trauma and burnout, which could harm their clients and themselves.

The study reveals that 80% of the MHPs experience high levels of vicarious trauma when working with children of high-conflict divorce and SPA survivors. The emotional toll of such trauma can manifest in various physical and mental health indicators, including tachycardia, nausea, rage, burnout, and emotional exhaustion. These symptoms affect the practitioners' well-being and ability to care for their clients effectively.

Additionally, the MHPs in these studies reported various personal and professional challenges when working in the SPA field. These challenges ranged from adverse physical and emotional health indicators to warnings and advice for peers in the field who work in private practice, group practice, social media, conferences, and Family Court. Some of the most significant challenges reported were threats from clients and their families, other PA experts and trolls, with one MHP explaining that they hire a bodyguard when speaking at SPA conferences.

Gender and Countertransference

Gender was highlighted when working with survivors. Data from the study recommends that MHPs consider the potential for transference and countertransference experiences, especially in cases where the practitioner may have shared a similar trauma experience with the client. Gender and countertransference during a session need to be considered carefully and empathically. The trauma literature emphasises the importance of practitioners and clients working together to establish a healthy therapeutic relationship. However, these studies report that a healthy therapeutic relationship with survivors may be challenging without clinically proven guidelines. These studies' MHP participants also recommend that if another practitioner experiences countertransference while listening to recounted trauma stories from clients, they must access clinical or peer supervision or private counselling from a supervisor/practitioner with extensive SPA knowledge and experience to prevent vicarious trauma.

SPA Field Challenges and Potential Harm

These studies report that working in the SPA field can be challenging and potentially harmful for MHPs. As Chapter Six outlines, MHPs may experience vicarious trauma, burnout, and even physical illnesses due to exposure to SPA. Another issue highlighted in the data is the potential physical health consequences of working with SPA clients, particularly in the Family Court system. For example, MHP3 warned that working in this area can be dangerous, and complaints from disgruntled clients can result in deregistration. This danger can cause stress and anxiety for practitioners, potentially leading to physical and mental health problems.

Professionals Fighting and Bullying Each Other

Practitioners and professionals are known to argue with each other within high-conflict divorce and SPA arenas. For example, the MHP and adult survivor study participants spoke openly about the arguing and mentioned instances of bullying and fighting within the culture of PA and SPA. Illustrations between the SPA professionals (researchers, psychiatrists, clinical psychologists, lawyers, and APs) included psychological abuse and professional attacks within the SPA and high-conflict divorce field.

The interviews revealed diverse experiences of bullying within the professional PA culture, with some MHPs reporting psychological abuse, choosing to maintain silence about PA work to protect their reputations, plagiarism, and professional attacks from other MHPs. Results also reported that the fighting is disturbing for the MHPs, survivors and family members experiencing SPA who are watching these behaviours and trying to work and heal in a highly volatile area simultaneously is difficult. For example, MHP9 cautioned that practitioners need to develop a plan to leave the field because other PA professionals may attack them, especially at conferences on PA, as they did with this MHP. Another MHP expressed concern about the fighting that has manifested between the 'expert' PA professionals and its negative impact on the MHPs and survivors who are watching these behaviours.

Recognising that bullying and fighting among professionals in the SPA field can negatively impact mentees, parents, and survivors seeking help. Such behaviours may also draw attention away from the critical issue of child abuse, which requires the expertise of SPA professionals. These studies recommend that experts in the PA field come together to address these concerns and work collaboratively to stop SPA. This collaboration may help to eliminate the fighting among the professionals and create a more supportive and safer environment for both MHPs and survivors. The MHPs in these studies warn that international PA experts might need to consider who is watching their behaviours, how it is holding up the work to solve SPA and how it affects those who look up to them. It is also crucial for them to consider the impact of their behaviour on their mentees, parents, and survivors who rely on their expertise to overcome the devastating effects.

The Effect on TLEs Regarding PA Professionals Fighting

On a personal note, the Researcher warns that the analogy of professional fighting among expert child psychological abuse professionals is akin to choosing between parents in a divorce, underscoring the challenging position professional individuals in the field with lived experience may find themselves in. In the context of SPA, where loyalty often becomes divided, aligning with one perspective over another can feel reminiscent of choosing sides in a familial dispute. As a researcher, MHP, and adult child survivor, the desire to remain impartial and inclusive of diverse viewpoints is paramount. Opting not to align with one side or another can be seen as a principled stance against bias and a commitment to the integrity of the field.

However, this decision can have professional consequences, as it may be perceived as controversial or even disloyal within certain circles. Refraining from taking sides may result in ostracisation or pushback from those who advocate for a specific approach or perspective. Nonetheless, maintaining objectivity and prioritising advancing knowledge and practice in the PA field is crucial for fostering meaningful progress and inclusivity. By refusing to engage in biased practices and remaining open to various viewpoints, you uphold the principles of fairness and integrity, even in the face of potential professional repercussions.

Inadequate Clinical Supervision

Another significant issue from the data was the difficulty for MHPs to find adequate clinical supervision. Many practitioners in these studies reported having to teach their supervisors about SPA and high-conflict divorce. Furthermore, the study reports that many supervisors do not have the necessary training and knowledge of SPA, resulting in inadequate support for the MHPs they supervise, which is a direct consequence of the dearth of availability regarding current SPA training. One MHP reported that their clinical supervisor experienced vicarious trauma from hearing about the practitioner's work with SPA clients, consequently withdrawing from the supervisory relationship and leaving the MHP with no supervisor.

Recommendations for SPA Training and Development

The final sub-theme of these studies explored the SPA training and development that MHPs recommend for colleagues who intend to work with survivors. Participants identified various training opportunities, including specialised courses in PA and SPA, trauma-informed care training, and attachment and bonding training. Other recommended training areas include family systems and structural therapy, training in the legal aspects of PA, SPA and SPAA, and courses focusing on self-care and managing and preventing vicarious trauma. These studies recommend that to address this issue, there needs to be a concerted effort to prioritise mental health research and the development of effective treatments for SPA.

Additionally, client dropout rates were identified as a concern for practitioners, with one in five clients leaving therapy before completion. Such a phenomenon can demoralise therapists, and the reasons for client dropout require further investigation and research. The Researcher questions whether the elevated client dropout rate is due to MHP's lack of experience regarding the identification and treatment of SPA, perhaps the cost is too high, or the toll of reliving the trauma in therapy may be too much if the survivor is not treated with care. Furthermore, the lack of awareness and training around SPA and its impact on survivors may perpetuate the stigmatisation and marginalisation of this population, adding to their reasons for not engaging in therapy. Practitioners who are not trained to recognise the signs and symptoms of SPA may inadvertently dismiss or pathologise their clients' experiences, leading to further trauma and harm. Therefore, MHPs must receive comprehensive training on SPA and its impact on survivors to ensure they provide competent and effective care to all their clients.

These studies' data reported why some MHPs might treat survivors without following best practice guidelines. For example, some MHPs believed they had sufficient knowledge and expertise to manage SPA cases, while others acknowledged the need for more training to fully understand SPA's complexity and severity. Moreover, the study revealed that some MHPs treat survivors despite lacking adequate training in this area or recognising the need for specialised training, as reported by their colleagues.

The failure to address the needs of this population perpetuates stigma and marginalisation, preserving the cycle of abuse and trauma. As a society, we must prioritise the needs of survivors and work to ensure they receive the care and support needed to heal and recover. However, it is not only the responsibility of practitioners to address and treat SPA. Others whom the adult survivor spoke to but were not referred to elsewhere to get the help they needed, such as general practitioners, psychiatrists, other psychologists, clinical psychotherapists, the police, teachers, family members, friends, and community members, also have a role to play. Professional community members can help prevent further harm and support healing by speaking up and taking action to support survivors.

Mental Health Field vs the Disability Field

The mental health field has fallen behind the disabilities field in researching and developing effective treatments for individuals with mental health challenges. This disparity is problematic as both fields deal with human suffering and well-being issues. The social model of disabilities has been adopted and significantly changed since the 1980s to combat how people with disabilities were socially constructed negatively. This change has led to significant progress in the field of disabilities, including establishing clear guidelines for treatments and preventative interventions. In contrast, the mental health field has not seen the same level of progress. The overall frequency of mental illness has not changed significantly within the past 30-40 years.

Furthermore, addressing the disparity between the disabilities and mental health fields is crucial to improving the well-being of individuals with mental health challenges. This change could involve public education campaigns about SPA to destigmatise mental health challenges and promote understanding of the impacts. This change could also foster increased collaboration between the fields of mental health and disabilities, facilitating the sharing of knowledge and resources, as these areas frequently overlap.

Therefore, society must take responsibility for addressing cultural issues that contribute to SPA and promote healthy family relationships to prevent the spread of this devastating phenomenon to future generations. As reported in these studies results, the intergenerational transmission of trauma resulting from SPA has significant implications for future generations. As reported by the MHP study participants, survivors often struggle with attachment, trust, and relationship-building issues, affecting their ability to form healthy relationships and parent their own children. This intergenerational trauma can result in a cycle of abuse, leading to the perpetuation of SPA and other forms of violence. However, there are also larger cultural issues beyond the immediate challenges SPA poses and its impact on mental health. The lack of research and formal training for working with survivors and the societal stigma associated with mental health challenges underscores the need for greater public awareness and education across many cultures and countries.

SPA Within African-American Communities

For example, these studies suggest that SPA is a recurring pattern in African-American communities, where fatherless homes are normalised, and SPA is used to maintain the adverse intergenerational cycles. This finding emphasises the need for culturally sensitive approaches to treating SPA and highlights the significance of addressing cultural issues in the broader societal context. Addressing cultural norms regarding SPA requires engaging with community leaders, advocates, and organisations to promote awareness and education about the harm of SPA and its impact on survivors and their communities. This may involve developing culturally sensitive approaches to addressing SPA, promoting policies supporting families and children, and challenging the cultural norms perpetuating abuse.

Prevention may also involve engaging with community leaders and advocates to promote awareness and education about the harm caused by SPA and its impact on survivors and their communities. Prevention may also involve the promotion of legal and policy reforms that protect survivors of SPA and hold perpetrators accountable for their actions. (Refer to Chapter Six, 'African-American Recommendations'). These studies report that ethically and culturally dealing with SPA requires a comprehensive approach that addresses the needs of survivors, promotes prevention efforts, and challenges the cultural norms perpetuating abuse. A trauma-informed and culturally sensitive approach is suggested to promote healing and social justice for survivors of SPA and their communities.

Concept of Meaningful Harm

The concept of meaningful harm refers to the potential harm that may result from certain actions or behaviours that significantly impact individuals or groups. In the context of SPA, the harm can be significant for both the child and the TP. Children subjected to SPA may experience significant harm, including losing a meaningful relationship with the TP, emotional trauma, and psychological distress. Furthermore, these studies report that the meaningful harm survivors have experienced as children manifests throughout their lives and returns later in life to be dealt with in therapeutic sessions. In addition, the study reports that the TP may experience harm, including a loss of parental rights, depression, and a breakdown in their relationship with their child.

MHPs must recognise the harm that can result from "winging it" themselves concerning treatment. As stated, this is a difficult time for MHPs until a protocol is developed, so they must be careful. Practitioners may overlook critical symptoms of SPA without clear guidelines, resulting in misdiagnosis or inadequate treatment. This can be particularly problematic in cases where the client has experienced significant trauma or from SPA throughout their life.

Legal and Regulatory Frameworks

These studies suggest that the government should intervene through legal and regulatory frameworks to address SPA, which will help limit the harm to children and TPs. An intervention may involve implementing laws and policies that protect the rights of children and survivors and promote healthy and meaningful relationships between parents and children. Additionally, the government may offer more funding to train MHPs so they are equipped to work with families experiencing SPA. By providing funding to educate and train more MHPs, families can start to rebuild and strengthen their relationships while promoting healthy communication and boundaries to prevent the lifelong trauma experienced by the survivors.

Stopping the practice of SPA can be challenging, mainly when there are limited consequences for those who engage in these behaviours. However, raising awareness and promoting education about PA, SPA, and SPAA's harmful effects can help prevent PABs and promote healthy and meaningful relationships among community members. These studies report that SPA can result in meaningful harm. Therefore, prevention efforts must address the root causes of SPA, including social, economic, and political factors contributing to family breakdown and the normalisation of abuse. Prevention may involve supporting healthy family relationships through education and community-based programs, promoting social policies that support families and children, and addressing systemic issues such as FDV, poverty, inequality, and discrimination.

The concept of harm is also relevant for MHPs working with survivors. Practitioners report experiencing vicarious trauma, compassion fatigue, and burnout from working with trauma survivors. The impact of SPA on survivors and their families can also be overwhelming and challenging to manage, requiring practitioners to take a trauma-informed and self-care approach to their work. This approach is important for MHPs who identify as TLEs. However, as explained, practice guidelines for MHPs regarding suggested self-care to prevent vicarious trauma have not yet been written. Therefore, these studies underscore the need for MHPs to receive proper training, ongoing professional development, and access to a set of standards of practice when working with survivors. Failing to do so may harm the clients and lead to significant professional and ethical consequences for the practitioners themselves.

How do we Ethically and Culturally Deal with SPA as a Society?

Ethically and culturally, dealing with SPA requires a nuanced and multifaceted approach that considers the unique needs and experiences of survivors of SPA and their communities. Recognising the harm it causes survivors and the intergenerational trauma it perpetuates is at the core of any ethical and cultural response. This level of recognition requires a commitment to promoting healing, prevention, and social justice through a trauma-informed and culturally sensitive lens.

Ethical Responsibility of the Mental Health Field

One higher-level argument that emerges from this research is the ethical responsibility of MHPs to recognise and address the trauma experienced by survivors. The findings suggest that many MHPs are not trained to identify the needs of this population or equipped with the tools to treat them effectively. This lack of recognition raises questions about the professional responsibility of the mental health field to address this gap in training and practice. The responsibility for addressing this issue falls on multiple parties, including mental health education programs, licensing boards, and professional organisations. Mental health education programs should ensure that their curricula include training on trauma-informed care and specifically address all forms of parental alienation as a form of trauma. Licensing Boards should require continuing education in trauma-informed care, and professional organisations should promote awareness and training for working with survivors. If we fail to address this problem, the impact on future generations could be significant.

Furthermore, without adequate support and treatment for survivors, they may struggle with mental health issues and potentially pass on unresolved trauma to their children. This perpetuates a cycle of trauma that can have intergenerational effects, underscoring the urgency of addressing this issue. Improving MHP training and awareness can help break this cycle and promote healing for individuals, families, and communities.

Causing Harm to a Client

These studies' results reveal another topic concerning the safety of MHPs who treat survivors. Suppose a practitioner causes harm to a client of SPA due to their lack of training. In that case, they may face significant professional and ethical consequences, including disciplinary action and legal repercussions. Various professional sanctions may be imposed on practitioners who harm a SPA client. For example, licensing Boards may investigate complaints of professional misconduct and impose sanctions such as revoking or suspending a practitioner's license, imposing fines, or requesting additional training or supervision. In some cases, practitioners may face civil lawsuits or criminal charges if they cause harm.

Risky Knowledge

The concept of risky knowledge refers to the potential harm that can result from certain types of knowledge, particularly in the context of marginalised or vulnerable populations. In the case of SPA, Chapter Five reports the risks of further harm as described by the survivors if MHPs do not have the appropriate training. These studies address the topic of risky knowledge by highlighting the potential harm that can result from inadequate treatment for SPA through survivors' perspectives. In addition, the study sheds light on the gaps in knowledge and practice to prevent further harm by providing a platform for MHPs to share their perspectives and experiences working with survivors.

Chapter Eight Conclusion

The findings from the MHPs in these studies indicate a lack of clear guidelines for treatments relating to survivors presenting for therapy. These studies report that MHPs adapt their treatment delivery intuitively, using a combination of non-specific and specific therapeutic interventions borrowed from other treatments. This lack of specificity highlights the need to develop an innovative psychosocial treatment model to address the biopsychosocial structure underlying mental health challenges in survivors of SPA. Developing a treatment framework also addresses the professional and ethical repercussions that MHPs face.

The imbalanced state of the mental health field, compared to other proactive human service fields, such as disabilities, also emphasises the need for more psychoeducation and research to restore the balance. The absence of formal training for MHPs working with survivors also creates a problem. The lack of clear treatment guidelines and the dangers and complexities associated with SPA complicate this issue. These studies recommend greater awareness and education around SPA for MHPs and the broader public. Failure to address the root cause of SPA can lead to misdiagnosis and inadequate treatment, perpetuating the intergenerational cycle of abuse.

It is clear from the data that practitioners in the field of SPA require a high level of complex training and support from their clinical supervisors to prevent negative consequences for both them and their clients. A lack of professional standards leaves MHPs vulnerable to complaints and deregistration due to not being held to specific standards within the SPA field. Furthermore, the data suggests that the challenges faced by MHPs working with SPA clients are compounded by the limited resources available on the training required for MHPs to work with survivors.

The shortage of trained professionals who can identify SPA suggests that MHPs work with survivors without realising it due to their disguised presentations (Gelinas, 1983) while also exposing them to stress and burnout. Moreover, the limited treatment options for SPA further contribute to the stress and frustration experienced by practitioners and survivors. Additionally, the specific phobias related to SPAA and the potential FDIOA, FDIOA and malingering and shared delusional disorder variants among the survivors have emerged as potentially significant clinical findings that MHPs need to be aware of as potential CITs.

The cultural issues surrounding SPA and its impact on future generations must also be addressed. The lack of research and formal training, combined with the complexities of SPA and SPAA, underscores the need for increased public awareness and education to prevent and treat SPA. Failure to address this issue now could lead to future generations suffering the same trauma, with the same lack of available resources for support and healing.

Overall, the data collected from MHPs working with survivors highlights the significant challenges and potential harm practitioners face in this field. The lack of professional training and a code of practice, combined with high caseloads and limited resources, leave practitioners vulnerable to vicarious trauma and burnout. These challenges affect not only the well-being of the practitioners but also their ability to provide effective care to their clients. Therefore, the SPA field must receive more attention, resources, and professional training to address the challenges practitioners, survivors, and their communities face.

Acknowledgement of a "Revolutionary Social Worker"

Please note: This acknowledgement will appear in Volumes One and Two as I believe the message is highly important. These studies have drawn upon and embraced the writings, ideas, and invitations put forward by Dr Dyann Ross (2020), a "Revolutionary Social Worker" who was also the Researcher's primary PhD supervisor. Dr Ross (2020) argues that MHPs should embrace the concept of "the person as revolutionary" (Ross, 2020, p. 8). Embracing the person in a revolutionary concept redefines the role of mental health professionals as being "nonviolent, loving and justice-seeking citizens of the world" (Ross, 2020, p.8). By promoting nonviolence, love, and justice in therapeutic relationships, professionals empower their clients to become agents of change in their lives and communities (Ross, 2020).

Furthermore, this approach allows mental health professionals to model and enable revolutionary practices within their professions, ultimately transforming how mental health care is provided and experienced (Ross, 2020). Furthermore, mental health professionals must be responsible for addressing power dynamics and structural inequalities that contribute to mental health disparities and act as strong advocates for vulnerable people who need support in this area (Ross, 2020).

Therefore, these studies recommend that MHPs and MH professionals take up Dr Ross's (2020) invitation to join together and embrace the following core values for revolutionary work as a collective: nurturing a compassionate vision, cultivating a sense of empowered optimism, championing innovative approaches, and upholding established nonviolent and equitable practices that have proven effective. Together, let us explore loving ecological and posthuman actions that challenge human-centeredness and prioritise alternative forms of knowledge and wisdom while fostering healing, resilience, and connection within therapeutic settings (Ross, 2020).

In conclusion, the study findings remind us that MHPs are critical in identifying and treating survivors. In addition, these studies have shed light on the significant challenges MHPs face when working with survivors. The results of these studies provide a valuable contribution to the existing literature and highlight the need for further research in mental and physical health symptomology combined to improve the understanding of SPA and its impact on survivors and their MHPs. These studies' findings will also contribute to developing a broader understanding of SPA's social, cultural, and political dimensions and its impact on survivors.

Future Research

Survivors

Further research proposed by these studies suggests that an in-depth investigation is necessary to comprehend the effects of the potentially new 'specific phobia-severe parental alienation, and abduction anxiety variant' (Price-Tobler, 2023) and the possible variant of FDIOA, and shared delusional disorder and the impact on adult child survivor populations. Future research should explore how sustained stress from SPA may weaken survivors' immune systems, potentially increasing their vulnerability to various health issues. Furthermore, future studies should examine the connections between SPA, physical health symptoms, and the interplay with mental well-being.

Moreover, it is vital to research the impact of SPA within African-American communities. This exploration will help gain insights into unique challenges, experiences, and support needs specific to these communities. In addition, it is essential to examine the reasons underlying SPA client dropout rates and how to improve client engagement in SPA services. Lastly, further research needs to be undertaken to develop, disseminate, and teach psychoeducational materials to survivors and the general community to enhance their understanding of SPA and promote more awareness within our community.

MHPs

Further research proposed by these studies for MHPs suggests that potential links between cancer and SPA among MHPs also need to be investigated. Further research is warranted to explore factors contributing to training, professional development and clinical supervision. Additionally, resolving the personal and professional differences among MHPs and other professionals is crucial so that the SPA field can move forward and stop child psychological abuse from continuing into the following generations.

A collaborative effort would promote practical interdisciplinary approaches, enhance patient care, and ensure ethical principles guide the delivery of SPA mental health services. By fostering open communication, mutual respect, and shared decision-making, MHPs and other professionals can work harmoniously to provide comprehensive and ethical care to child and adult survivors while not contributing to further harm.

Finally, by recognising the interchange between physical and mental health, professionals and caregivers can provide more comprehensive support to help mitigate the potential long-term effects of SPA on child and adult overall health. By delving into the complex relationship between physical and mental health, researchers can enhance our understanding of the potential consequences experienced by all people affected by SPA.

Contributions of Study

These studies significantly contribute to the existing literature by offering valuable insights into the perspectives and challenges survivors and MHPs face when working together. The findings highlight the urgent need for a clinically tested treatment protocol and specialised training to equip MHPs, their clinical supervisors and medical professionals with the necessary knowledge and skills to identify and effectively address SPA-related mental and physical health issues with their clients. Moreover, 100% of the study participants acknowledge the misunderstood complexity of SPA and suggest developing a multifaceted collaborative treatment approach. Finally, these findings underscore the importance of continued research and the need for combined concerted efforts to improve the support and treatment provided to ALL community members affected by SPA.

Final Note from the Author Regarding Peer Review and Publishing in Book Form

Having undergone rigorous peer review by academic supervisors and internal and external examiners before reaching the conferment stage, my PhD ensures my work's academic rigour and credibility. Thus, anyone suggesting that the majority of the content in Volume One and Two is not peer-reviewed may not have a strong argument. This academic foundation provides a solid platform for navigating the complexities of research in the pioneering realm of adult survivors of child psychological abuse research and the dedicated mental health practitioners who navigate this terrain; conflict is not just prevalent; it is ubiquitous. Parents are embroiled in battles for custody, experts spar over research methodologies, terminologies, and affiliations, while the children and adult survivors observe from the shadows. However, this status quo is undergoing a transformative shift.

As a recent PhD recipient immersed in the pioneering field of SPA research and therapeutic intervention, I confront a formidable hurdle: the exorbitant publishing fees that now loom ominously over academia. Even with the involvement of PhD supervisors and PA experts in co-authoring publications from the twin PhD, we faced hurdles in getting them published, indicating the complexity and difficulties in navigating the process. I am now at a crossroads no longer shielded by the read-and-publish agreements afforded to PhD candidates.

By opting for a book format, I could present my findings comprehensively, weaving together diverse content and insights that the limitations of journal articles might have constrained. Moreover, books offer a longer shelf life, ensuring that my research remains accessible and relevant to academic and practitioner audiences for years to come. This approach aligns with my goal of making meaningful contributions to the field while navigating the challenges of limited resources. Additionally, the expedited publication process of a book allows for quicker dissemination of crucial information, potentially saving lives by providing timely insights for mental health practitioners to understand better and support adult survivors of trauma.

Could this be the harbinger of a new era in academic publishing? A paradigm shift where scholars reclaim control over their narratives, unencumbered by prohibitive publishing fees? The resonance of this decision extends far beyond my individual circumstances—it signals a rallying cry for academics worldwide who refuse to be shackled by the confines of traditional publishing models. It's a clarion call for innovation, inclusivity, and accessibility in scholarly dissemination. I dream of a future where knowledge knows no bounds and voices previously marginalised find their rightful place in the academic discourse.

Finally, the phrase "the children are coming" has evolved into "the adult children are here." We are speaking up, advocating that nothing is written about us without our input. We also assert that conferences addressing our trauma must include representation from lived-experience adult survivors, with a requirement that at least 50% of speakers have lived experience. Our hashtag is #NothingAboutUsWithoutUs #NAUWOU.

Additionally, I extend a warm invitation for you to consult with adult survivors on academic literature pertaining to our experiences before publication. Your collaboration ensures that our narratives are accurately represented, reflecting the diverse perspectives within our community. We welcome your engagement and value your commitment to understanding our journey. Please feel free to reach out; we can create a more inclusive and empathetic discourse together. Remember, it is not just about collecting data from us; it is about checking in with us before publishing. Additionally, if you consult us professionally, consider including us as named authors on research papers, honouring our contribution and expertise.

Gratitude for the MHP Study Cohort

To the Mental Health Practitioners who contributed to this thesis:
Your invaluable contributions have been deeply inspiring and have enriched this work immeasurably. Your dedication to the field of mental health, in particular child survivors of psychological abuse, makes you warriors in a frontline battle, navigating an area with limited knowledge about what you must learn and practice to work with survivors. You confront difficult and dangerous personality types in a litigious field worth 70 billion dollars a year, and your resilience and commitment to caring for the broken system's victims are commendable. Thank you for your unwavering commitment and for sharing your expertise. Your involvement has strengthened this research and fostered a community of support and collaboration in our collective pursuit of improving mental health care.

As we continue on this journey, it is my hope that this research will serve as a foundation for implementing strategies to assist practitioners in preventing vicarious trauma, recognising and addressing the physical and mental health effects that may arise, and supporting their ongoing professional development. Moreover, by fostering understanding within organisations that work with this vulnerable population, we can create environments conducive to the well-being of practitioners and those they serve. You are all MY heroes.

A Message for MHPs Working in PA

For those who will be working with adult trauma survivors, may this body of work serve as a guiding light, offering insights and perspectives to aid in your compassionate and effective care. Within these pages, I offer knowledge and a source of hope—a gentle reminder of the transformative potential within your hands. Each new CIT learned, each innovative approach embraced, holds the potential to bring solace and save lives. Your ongoing commitment to growth underscores your profound impact on those you serve.

As we navigate the intricate landscape of trauma, particularly among adult child survivors of psychological abuse, I encourage you to explore the sample lists of suggested professional development subjects, modalities and holistic ideas provided within Volumes One and Two. These resources offer invaluable insights to enrich your practice and deepen your understanding when working with this vulnerable population. I am also including the reference list for the PhD in both volumes so that you can look up and read about others who have gone before us in this specialised field.

Look forward to Volume Three, where a comprehensive treatment framework awaits. May this forthcoming resource ignite your passion and guide your journey to greater heights in the noble pursuit of healing.

With sincere appreciation for your unwavering dedication and heartfelt gratitude,

Dr. Alyse Price-Tobler (PhD)

References

ACES Too High News. (2020, May 20). Retrieved from ACES Too High: https://acestoohigh.com/got-your-ace-score/

Adams, S. A., & Riggs, S. A. (2008). An exploratory study of vicarious trauma among therapist trainees. *Training and Education in Professional Psychology, 2*(1), 26-34. doi:https://doi-org.ezproxy.usc.edu.au/10.1037/1931-3918.2.1.26

Ahrens, C. E., Stansell, J., & Jennings, A. (2010). To Tell or Not to Tell: The Impact of Disclosure on Sexual Assault Survivors' Recovery. *Violence and Victims, 25*(5), 631-648. Retrieved February February 11, 2023, 2023, from https://www.proquest.com/docview/817785178?accountid=28745&parentSessionId=lpvSLwjyUL7haPMlMTSKxRf1N5x8WuCHx-rZf1IUOlbU%3D&pq-origsite=primo

Alaggia, R. (2010, February). An Ecological Analysis of Child Sexual Abuse Disclosure: Considerations for Child and Adolescent Mental Health. *Journal of the Canadian Academy of Child and Adolescent Psychiatry, 19*(1), 23-39. Retrieved February 11, 2023, from https://www.ncbi.nlm.nih.gov/pmc/articles/PMC2809444/

Alder, C., & Polk, K. (2001). *Child Victims of Homicide.* Cambridge: Cambridge University Press.

Alexander, P. C. (2015). *Intergenerational Cycles of Trauma and Violence. An Attachment and Family Systems Perspective* (1 ed.). New York, NY, America: W.W Norton & Company Inc.

Alvarez, M., & Turner, C. (ND). *About Us.* Retrieved from Resetting the Family: https://www.resetting-the-family.com/

American Cancer Society. (2023). *Cancer Clusters.* Retrieved June 30, 2023, from American Cancer Society: https://www.cancer.org/cancer/risk-prevention/understanding-cancer-risk/cancer-clusters.html

American Cancer Society. (2023, June 30). *Do X-rays and Gamma Rays Cause Cancer?* Retrieved 2023, from American Cancer Society: https://www.cancer.org/cancer/risk-prevention/radiation-exposure/x-rays-gamma-rays/do-xrays-and-gamma-rays-cause-cancer.html

American Psychiatric Association. (2013). *Diagnostic and Statistical Manual of Mental Disorders DSM-5* (5 ed.). Arlington, VA, USA: American Psychiatric Publishing. Retrieved October 238, 2021

American Psychiatric Association. (2013). *Diagnostics and Statistical Manual of Mental Disorders* (5 ed.). Arlington, Virginia, America: American Psychiatric Publishing. Retrieved November 1, 2020

American Psychological Association. (2020). *APA Dictionary of Psychology.* Retrieved June 23, 2020, from American Psychological Association: https://dictionary.apa.org/psychodynamic-theory

American Psychological Association. (2021, June). *Carl Rogers, PhD. 1947 APA President.* Retrieved April 10, 2023, from American Psychological Association: https://www.apa.org/about/governance/president/carl-r-rogers

Anand, K. S., & Dhikav, V. (2012, Oct-Dec). Hippocampus in health and disease: An overview. *Annals of Indian Academy of Neurology, 15*(4), 239-246. doi: 10.4103/0972-2327.104323

Anderson, C. A., & Bushman, B. J. (2002, February 1). Human Aggression. *Annual Review of Psychology, 53*(1), 27-51. doi:10.1146/annurev.psych.53.100901.135231

Andrews, T. (2012). What is Social Constructionism? *The Grounded Theory Review, 11*(1), 39-46. Retrieved March 12, 2023, from https://web-p-ebscohost-com.ezproxy.usc.edu.au/ehost/pdfviewer/pdfviewer?vid=1&sid=e45494c5-4762-4104-9622-f384ee8528f9%40redis

Arksey, H., & O'Malley, L. (2003). Scoping studies: towards a methodological framework. *International Journal of Social Research Methodology, 8*(1), 19-32. doi:doi-org.ezproxy.usc.edu.au/10.1080/1364557032000119616

Australian Government. (2019, November 27). *Marriages and Divorces, Australia.* Retrieved July 26, 2021, from Australian Bureau of Statistics: https://www.abs.gov.au/statistics/people/people-and-communities/marriages-and-divorces-australia/latest-release

Australian Government. (2022, November 17). *What is family and domestic violence?* Retrieved January 14, 2023, from Services Australia:

https://www.servicesaustralia.gov.au/what-family-and-domestic-violence?context=60033

Australian Human Rights Commission. (1997). *Bringing Them Home.* Canberra: Commonwealth of Australia. Retrieved January 17, 2021, from https://humanrights.gov.au/our-work/bringing-them-home-report-1997

Australian Institute of Aboriginal and Torres Strait Islander Studies. (2012). *Guidelines for Ethical Research in Australian Indigenous Studies.* AIATSIS. Australian Institute of Aboriginal and Torres Strait Islander Studies. Retrieved August 17, 2023, from https://aiatsis.gov.au/sites/default/files/2020-09/gerais.pdf

Australian Institute of Health and Welfare. (2018-2019, March 18). *Child Protection Australia 2018-19: children in the child protection system.* Retrieved February 9, 2021, from Australian Institute of Health and Welfare: https://www.aihw.gov.au/reports/child-protection/child-protection-australia-children-in-the-child-protection-system/contents/children-in-substantiated-cases-of-abuse-or-neglect

Bahtiyar, S., Karaca, K. G., Henckens, M. J., & Roozendaal, B. (2020, October). Norepinephrine and glucocorticoid effects on the brain mechanisms underlying memory accuracy and generalization. *Molecular and Cellular Neuroscience, 108*, 1-10. doi:https://doi.org/10.1016/j.mcn.2020.103537

Baker, A. (1994, January). The cult of parenthood: A qualitative study of parental alienation. *Cultic Studies Review, 4*(1), 20. Retrieved February 15, 2021, from Research Gate: https://www.researchgate.net/publication/228344114_The_cult_of_parenthood_A_qualitative_study_of_parental_alienation

Baker, A. J. (2006). Patterns of Parental Alienation Syndrome: A Qualitative Study of Adults Who were Alienated from a Parent as a Child. *American Journal of Family Therapy, 34*(1), 63-78. doi:10.1080/01926180500301444

Baker, A. J. (2007). *Adult Children of Parental Alienation Syndrome. Breaking the Ties that Bind.* New York, New York, USA: W.W Norton & Company. Retrieved November 7, 2020

Baker, A. J. (2007). *Adult Children of Parental Alienation Syndrome. Breaking the Ties that Bind.* New York, New York, USA: W.W Norton & Company. Retrieved November 7, 2020

Baker, A. J., & Chambers, J. (2011, January 7). Adult Recall of Childhood Exposure to Parental Conflict: Unpacking the Black Box of Parental

Alienation. *Journal of Divorce and Remarriage, 52*(1), 55-76. doi:10.108
0/10502556.2011.534396

Baker, A. J., & Fine, P. R. (2014). *Surviving Parental Alienation: A Journey of Hope and Healing.* Lanham, Maryland, USA: Rowman & Littlefield.

Baker, A. J., & Schneiderman, M. (2015). Bonded to the Abuser. How victims make sense of the abuse. London, England: Rowman & Littlefield.

Baker, A. J., & Verrocchio, C. (2014, December 25). Parental Bonding and Parental Alienation as Correlates of Psychological Maltreatment in Adults in Intact and Non-intact Families. *Journal of Child and Family Studies, 24,* 3047-3057. doi:DOI 10.1007/s10826-014-0108-0

Baker, A. J., & Verrocchio, M. C. (2013, November 13). Italian College Student-Reported Childhood Exposure to Parental Alienation: Correlates With Well-Being. *Journal of Divorce & Remarriage, 54*(8), 609-628. doi:10.10 80/10502556.2013.837714

Baker, A. J., Fine, P. R., & Lacheen-Baker, A. (2020). *Restoring Family Connections.* Lanham, Maryland, USA: Rowman & Littlefield. Retrieved January 28, 2022

Barnett, J. E., & Coffman, C. (2015, June). *Termination and Abandonment. A Proactive Approach to Ethical Practice.* Retrieved June 7, 2021, from Society for the Advancement of Psychotherapy: www.society-forpsychotherapy.org/termination-and-abandonment-a-proactive-approach-to-ethical-practice

Bentley, C., & Matthewson, M. (2020). The Not-Forgotten Child: Alienated Adult Children's Experience of Parental Alienation. *The American Journal of Family Therapy, 48*(5), 509-529. doi:https://www.tandfonline.com/doi/full/10.1080/01926187.2020.1775531

Bergen, R. K. (1993). Interviewing survivors of marital rape: Doing feminist research on sensitive topics. In *Researching Sensitive Topics* (pp. 197-211). Newbury Park, California, USA: Sage.

Berkowitz, A. R. (n.d). *Parental Alienation Syndrome.* Retrieved June 26, 2021, from Dr Alice R Berkowitz: https://www.draliceberkowitz.com/alienation

Bernet, W. (2008, October 13). Parental Alienation Disorder and DSM-V. *The American Journal of Family Therapy, 36*(5), 349-366. doi:https://doi.org/10.1080/01926180802405513

Bernet, W. (2010). *Parental Alienation, DSM-5, and ICD-11.* Springfield, Illinois, USA: Charles C Thomas.

Blakely, L. (2022, February 21). Learning to Become a More Ethically Focused Practitioner Researcher: Developing Through the Research Ethics Process. *Ethics and Social Welfare, 16*(3), 322-331. doi:https://doi-org.ezproxy.usc.edu.au/10.1080/17496535.2022.2033397

Boonzaier, F., & de la Rey, C. (2004, September 1). Woman Abuse: The Construction of Gender in Women and Men's Narratives of Violence. *South African Journal of Psychology, 34*(3), 443-463. doi:https://doi-org.ezproxy.usc.edu.au/10.1177/008124630403400307

Boswell, E., & Babchuk, W. (2022). Philosophical and theoretical underpinnings of qualitative research. In *INTERNATIONAL ENCYLOPEDIA OF EDUCATION* (pp. 1-13). Lincoln, NE, America. doi:DOI:10.1016/b978-0-12-818630-5.11001-2

Bourget, D., Grace, J., & Whitehurst, L. (2007, March). A Review of Maternal and Paternal Filicide. *The Journal of the American Academy of Psychiatry and the Law, 35*(1), 74-82. Retrieved May 28, 2023, from https://jaapl.org/content/35/1/74.long

Bourne, E. J. (1998). *Overcoming Specific Phobia. A Hierarchy and Exposure-Based Protocol for the Treatment of All Specific Phobias.* (C. Honeychurch, Ed.) Oakland, California, United States: Publisher's West Group.

Bowlby, J. (1980). *Loss, Sadness and Depression* (Vol. 3). New York, New York, America: The Travistock Institute of Human Resources.

Bowlby, J. (1988). *A Secure Base: Clinical Applications of Attachment Theory.* New York: Brunner-Routledge.

Boyatzis, R. E. (1998). *Transforming Qualitative Information.* London: SAGE Publications.

Braun, V., & Clarke, V. (2006). Using thematic analysis in psychology. *Qualitative Research in Psychology, 3*(2), 77-101. doi:10.1191/1478088706qp063oa

Braun, V., & Clarke, V. (2014, October 16). What can "thematic analysis" offer health and wellbeing researchers? *International Journal of Qualitative Studies in Health and Well-being, 9*(10), 1-3. doi:10.3402/qhw.v9.26152

Briere, J. N. (1992). *Child Abuse Trauma.* Southern California, USA: Sage Publications Inc.

Briere, J., & Runtz, M. (1987). Post Sexual Abuse Trauma: Data and Implications for Clinical Practice. *Journal of Interpersonal Violence, 2*(4), 376-379. doi:https://doi-org.ezproxy.usc.edu.au/10.1177/088626058700200403

Briere, J., & Runtz, M. (1993, September 1). Childhood Sexual Abuse Long term Sequelae and Implications for Psychological Assessment. *Journal of Interpersonal Violence, 8*(3), 312-330. doi:https://doi-org.ezproxy.usc.edu.au/10.1177/088626093008003002

Briere, J., & Spinazzola, J. (2005). Phenomenology and psychological assessment of complex trauma states. *Journal of Traumatic Stress, 18*(5), 401-412. doi:DOI:10.1002/jts.20048

Britannica Dictionary. (2023). *Homicide-Law*. Retrieved from Britannica: https://www.britannica.com/biography/Richard-Ramirez

Brown, D. P., & Elliot, D. S. (2016). *Attachment Disturbances in Adults. Treatment for Comprehensive Repair* (Vol. One). New York, New York, America: W W Norton and Company, Inc. Retrieved October 8, 2022

Brown, T., Tyson, D., & Arias, P. F. (2014, April 16). Filicide and Parental Separation and Divorce. *Child Abuse Review. Association of Child Protection Professionals, 23*, 79-88. doi:10.1002/car.2327

Bruce, T. J., & Sanderson, W. C. (1998). *Specific Phobias, Clinical Applications of Evidence Based Psychotherapy*. (R. D. Hack, Ed.) Montebello, NY, United States: Book-mart Press.

Bryant, A., & Charmaz, K. (2007). *The SAGE Handbook of Grounded Theory*. London: SAGE Publications Ltd.

Burr, V. (2003). *Social Constructionism* (2 ed.). New York, NY, USA: Routledge.

Butz, M. R., & Evans, F. (2019). Factitious Disorder by Proxy, Parent Alienation, and the Argument for Interrelated Multidimensional Diagnoses. *Professional Psychology: Research and Practice, 50*(6), 364-375. doi:https://doi-org.ezproxy.usc.edu.au/10.1037/pro0000250

Cahill, L., & Alkire, M. (2003, March). Epinephrine enhancement of human memory consolidation: Interaction with arousal at encoding. *Neurobiology of Learning and Memory, 79*(2), 194-198. doi:https://doi.org/10.1016/S1074-7427(02)00036-9

Campbell, C., & Clarke, M. (2019, July 18). The 'Worker-Researcher': Introducing a new interview dynamic. *Qualitative Research in Psychology, 19*(2), 405-423. doi:https://doi-org.ezproxy.usc.edu.au/10.1080/14780887.2019.1644408

Canadian Center for Occupational Health and Safety. (2023, June 13). *Occupational Cancer*. Retrieved June 30, 2023, from Canadian Center

for Occupational Health and Safety: https://www.ccohs.ca/oshanswers/
diseases/cancer/occupational_cancer.html#:~:text=The%20most%20
common%20types%20of,cancer%2C%20bladder%20cancer%20and%20
mesothelioma.&text=*%20In%20general%2C%20the%20overall%20
attributable,risk%20may%20be%20around%2090%25.

Carpenter, L. L., Tyrka, A. R., Ross, N. S., Khoury, L., Anderson, G. M., & Price,
L. H. (2009, July 1). Effect of Childhood Emotional Abuse and Age on
Cortisol Responsivity in Adulthood. *Biological Psychiatry, 66*(1), 69-75.
doi:https://doi.org/10.1016/j.biopsych.2009.02.030

Cashmore, J., & Shackel, R. (2013, January). *The long-term effects of child
sexual abuse.* Retrieved May 19, 2023, from Australian Government.
Australian Institue of Family Studies: https://aifs.gov.au/resources/
policy-and-practice-papers/long-term-effects-child-sexual-abuse

Centers for Disease Control and Prevention. (2019). *Marriage and Divorce.*
Retrieved July 26, 2021, from National Centers for Disease Control and
Prevention: https://www.cdc.gov/nchs/fastats/marriage-divorce.htm

Centers for Disease Control and Prevention. (2020, April 20). *Violence
Prevention.* Retrieved February 15, 2021, from Centers for Disease
Control and Prevention: https://www.cdc.gov/violenceprevention/aces/
fastfact.html?CDC_AA_refVal=https%3A%2F%2Fwww.cdc.gov%2Fvi-
olenceprevention%2Facestudy%2Ffastfact.html

Chamberlin, J. (2015, April). Are your clients leaving too soon? *American
Psychological Association, 46*(4), 1-5. Retrieved December 4, 2022, from
https://www.apa.org/monitor/2015/04/clients

Charmaz, K. (2014). *Constructing Grounded Theory* (2 ed.). Sage Publications.

Childress, C. (2014, December 4). Treatment of Attachment-Based "Parental
Alienation". *CalSouthern Psychology.* California, America. Retrieved
June 17, 2021, from https://www.youtube.com/watch?v=ezBJ3954mKw

Childress, C. (2024, May 6). Sunday Coffee w/ Dr. Childress: Using Euphemism
for Child Abuse Hides the Child Abuse. *Video.* California, USA: You
Tube. Retrieved May 5, 2024, from https://www.youtube.com/channel/
UCV-OK9_OFd3BgBWgB0ccw4w/about

Childress, C. A. (2015). *Foundations.* Claremont, California, America: Oaksong
Press. Retrieved October 31, 2020

Childress, C. A. (2022). *Child Custody Evaluations*. Retrieved January 30, 2022, from Dr Craig A Childress: https://drcachildress.org/custom-page/6-child-custody-evaluations/

Childress, C. A. (2022). *The Office of Dr C.A. Childress*. Retrieved January 30, 2022, from Dr C.A Childress: https://drcachildress.org/

Chorpita, B. F., Albano, A., & Barlow, D. H. (2010, June 7). Child Anxiety Sensitivity Index: Considerations for Children with Anxiety Disorders. *Journal of Clinical Child Psychology, 25*(1), 77-82. doi:https://doi-org.ezproxy.usc.edu.au/10.1207/s15374424jccp2501_9

Clawar, S. S., & Rivlin, B. V. (2014). *Children Held Hostage: Identifying Brainwashed Children, Presenting a Case, and Crafting Solutions*. Chicago, Illinois, America: American Bar Association.

Cleary, R., & Armour, C. (2022, July 29). Exploring the role of practitioner lived experience of mental health issues in counselling and psychotherapy. *Counselling and Psychotherapy Research, 22*(4), 1100-1111. doi:https://doi.org/10.1002/capr.12569

Cleary, R., & Armour, C. (2022, July 29). Exploring the role of practitioner lived experience of mental health issues in counselling and psychotherapy. *Counselling and Psychotherapy Research, 22*(4), 1100-1111. doi: https://doi.org/10.1002/capr.12569

Coan, J. A. (2008). *Toward a neuroscience of attachment: Theory, research, and clinical applications*. New York, America: Guildford.

Collins Dictionary. (2023). *Definition of familicide*. Retrieved January 14, 2023, from Collins Dictionary: https://www.collinsdictionary.com/dictionary/english/familicide

Collins-Mrakas, A. (2004). *Guidelines for Conducting Research with People who are Homeless*. Retrieved Nov 13, 2015, from York University: http://www.yorku.ca/research/documents/2010Guidelines%20-%20Research%20with%20People%20who%20are%20Homeless.doc

Conscious Co-Parenting Institute. (2022). *Conscious Co-Parenting Institute Hits New Milestone During Pandemic*. Retrieved January 13, 2022, from Conscious Co-Parenting Institute: https://www.consciousco-parentinginstitute.com/conscious-co-parenting-institute-hits-new-milestone-during-pandemic/

Conscious Co-Parenting Institute. (2022). *Our Mission*. Retrieved January 13, 2022, from Conscious Co-Parenting Institute: https://www.consciousco-parentinginstitute.com/

Cook, J. M., Dinnen, S., Rehman, O., Bufka, L., & Courtois, C. (2011). Responses of a sample of practicing psychologists to questions about clinical work with trauma and interest in specialized training. *Psychological Trauma: Theory, Research, Practice, and Policy, 3*(3), 253-257. doi: https://doi.org/10.1037/a0025048

Cooper, K. M., Gin, L. E., & Brownell, S. E. (2020, June 4). Depression as a concealable stigmatized identity: what influences whether students conceal or reveal their depression in undergraduate research experiences? *International Journal of Stem Education, 7*(27). doi:https://doi.org/10.1186/s40594-020-00216-5

Cotter, G. (2023, January 13). (A. M.-A. Price-Tobler, Interviewer) Wollongong, NSW, Australia.

Courtois, C. A. (2004). Complex Trauma, Complex Reactions: Assessment and Treatment. *Psychotherapy: Theory, Research, Practice, Training, 41*(4), 412-425. doi:http://dx.doi.org.ezproxy.usc.edu.au:2048/10.1037/0033-3204.41.4.412

Courtois, C. A., & Ford, J. D. (2009). *Treating complex traumatic stress disorders: An evidence-based guide*. The Guildford Press.

Cresswell, J. W. (2003). *Research Design: Qualitative, Quantitative, and Mixed Methods Approaches*. SAGE Publications Ltd.

Cresswell, J. W., & Poth, C. N. (2017). *Qualitative Inquiry and Research Design. Choosing Among Five Approaches*. Thousand Oaks, California, America: Sage Publications.

Critchfield, K. L., & Benjamin, L. S. (2008). Internalized representations of early interpersonal experience and adult relationships: a test of copy process theory in clinical and non-clinical settings. *Psychiatry, Interpersonal & Biological Processes, 71*(1), 71-92. doi:10.1521/psyc.2008.71.1.71

Cromby, J. (1999). *What's wrong with social constructionism*. Leics, England, UK: Loughborough University. Retrieved April 3, 2023, from https://www.academia.edu/767706/Whats_wrong_with_social_constructionism

Darnall, D. (1998). *Divorce Casualties. Protecting your Children From Parental Alienation*. Lanham, Maryland, USA: Taylor Trade Publishing. Retrieved January 9, 2021

Das, C. (2016). *British-Indian Adult Children of Divorce* (Vol. 1). New York, NY, USA: Ashgate Publishing.

Das, C. (2016). *British-Indian Adult Children of Divorce. Context, Impact and Coping.* (2 ed.). New York, NY, USA: Routledge Publishing.

Davis, N. (2022). *The Joy of Living Our Heart's Knowing and Imagining.* (P. deLaney, Ed.) Katoomba, NSW, Australia: Lifeflow Education. Retrieved May 12, 2024

De Bellis, M. D. (2001, September 27). Developmental traumatology: The psychobiological development of maltreated children and its implications for research, treatment, and policy. *Development and Psychopathology, 13*(3), 539-564. doi: https://doi.org/10.1017/S0954579401003078

De Quervain, D., Schwabe, L., & Roozendaal, B. (2017, January). Stress, glucocorticoids and memory: implications for treating fear-related disorders. *Nature Reviews. Neuroscience, 18*(1), 7-19. doi:DOI:10.1038/nrn.2016.155

Debowska, A., Boduszek, D., & Dhingra, K. (2015, March-April). Victim, perpetrator, and offense characteristics in filicide and filicide–suicide. *Aggression and Violent Behaviour, 21*, 113-124. doi:https://doi.org/10.1016/j.avb.2015.01.011

Denzin, N. K., & Lincoln, Y. S. (2000). *Handbook of Qualitative Research* (2 ed., Vol. 2). London: SAGE publications.

Devinsky, O. (2000). Right Cerebral Hemisphere Dominance for a Sense of Corporeal and Emotional Self. *Epilepsy & Behavior, 1*(1), 60-73. doi:https://doi.org/10.1006/ebeh.2000.0025

Downey, J. C., Gudmunson, C. G., Pang, Y. C., & Lee, K. (2017, February 8). Adverse Childhood Experiences Affect Health Risk Behaviors and Chronic Health of Iowans. *Journal of Family Violence, 32*, 557-564. doi:https://doi-org.ezproxy.usc.edu.au/10.1007/s10896-017-9909-4

DuMont, K. A., Widom, C. S., & Czaja, S. J. (2007). Predictors of resilience in abused and neglected children grown-up: The role of individual and neighborhood characteristics. *Child Abuse & Neglect, 31*(3), 255-274. doi:https://doi.org/10.1016/j.chiabu.2005.11.015

Eeny Meeny Miny Mo Foundation. (n.d.). *What is Parental Alienation.* Retrieved July 30, 2021, from Eeny Meeny Miny Mo Foundation: https://emmm.org.au/parental-alienation

Egeland, B., Jacobvitz, D., & Sroufe, A. L. (1988, August 1). Breaking the cycle of abuse. *Society for Research in Child Development, 59*(4), 1080-1088. doi:10.2307/1130274

Ellis, A. E., Gold, S. N., Courtois, C., Araujo, K., & Quinones, M. (2019). Supervising Trauma Treatment: The Contextual Trauma Treatment Model Applied to Supervision. *Practice Innovations, 4*(3), 166-181. doi:https://doi.org/10.1037/pri0000095

Elshaikh, E. M. (n.d). *Standing on the Shoulders of Invisible Giants*. Retrieved August 4, 2023, from Khan Academy: https://www.khanacademy.org/humanities/big-history-project/big-bang/how-did-big-bang-change/a/standing-on-the-shoulders-of-invisible-giants

Erel, D. (2022). *Handling Parental Alienation as a Medical Emergency*. Retrieved January 13, 2022, from Parental Alienation Study Group: https://pasg.info/app/uploads/2019/07/Erel_Medical_Emergency_2019_11.pdf

Fares, R., Najem, R., Hallit, S., Pelissolo, A., Haddad, G., & Naja, W. J. (2023, April 23). Parental alienation in Lebanon: a case report. *Journal of Medical Case Reports, 17*(1), 1-12. doi:doi: 10.1186/s13256-023-03911-3

Felitti, V. J., Anda, R. F., Nordenberg, D., Williamson, D. F., Spitz, A. M., Edwards, V., . . . Marks, J. S. (1998). Relationship of Childhood Abuse and Household Dysfunction to Many of the Leading Causes of Death in Adults. *American Journal of Preventative Medicine, 14*(4), 245-258. doi:https://doi.org/10.1016/S0749-3797(98)00017-8

Fidler, B. J., & Bala, N. (2010, January 15). Children Resisting Postseparation Contact With a Parent: Concepts, Controversies, and Conundrums. *Family Court Review. An Interdisciplinary Journal, 48*(1). doi:https://doi-org.ezproxy.usc.edu.au/10.1111/j.1744-1617.2009.01287.x

Fidler, B., Bala, N., & Saini, M. (2012). *Children Who Resist PostSeparation Parental Contact: A Different Approach For Legal and Mental Health Professionals*. New York: Oxford University Press.

Fine, M., Weis, L., Weseen, S., & Wong, L. (2000). *For Whom? Qualitative research, representations, and social responsibilities*. Thousand Oaks, California, USA: Sage.

Finkelhor, D., & Browne, A. (1985). THE TRAUMATIC IMPACT OF CHILD SEXUAL ABUSE: A Conceptualization. *American Journal of*

Orthopsychiatry, 55(4), 530-541. doi:http://dx.doi.org.ezproxy.usc.edu.
au:2048/10.1111/j.1939-0025.1985.tb02703.x

Finlay, L. (2011). *Phenomenology for Therapists Researching the Lived World*
(Vol. 1). Chichester, West Sussex, United Kingdom: John Wiley & Sons
Ltd.

Flaskerud, J. H., & Winslow, B. W. (2010, March 10). Vulnerable Populations
and Ultimate Responsibility. *Issues in Mental Health Nursing, 31*(4),
298-299. doi:https://doi.org/10.3109/01612840903308556

Fonagy, P., & Luyten, P. (2019, September 9). Fidelity vs. flexibility in the
implementation of psychotherapies: time to move on. *World Psychiatry,
18*(3), 270-271. doi: https://doi.org/10.1002/wps.20657

Foucault, M. (1988). *Technologies of the Self.* (P. H. Hutton, H. Gutman, &
L. H. Martin, Eds.) University of Vermont, Vermont, USA.

Galanena, C. (2019). Presentation-child abuse. (pp. 1-4). Campbelltown:
Western Sydney University. Retrieved December 5, 2022, from https://
www.studocu.com/en-au/document/western-sydney-university/
child-abuse-as-a-social-issue/presentation-child-abuse/8770829

Galbin, A. (2014, December). An introduction to social constructionism. *Social
Research Reports, 26*, 82-92. Retrieved March 31, 2023, from https://
www.proquest.com/docview/1752382689?accountid=28745&parent-
SessionId=0GmTKmvk5OFYnCRHiE9IRFo1ammo4Tj6wnZQt8Qlz-
t8%3D&pq-origsite=primo

Garber, B. D. (2004). Therapist Alienation: Foreseeing and Forestalling Third-
Party Dynamics Undermining Psychotherapy With Children of Conflicted
Caregivers. *Professional Psychology: Research and Practice, 35*(4), 357-
363. doi:doi:10.1037/0735-7028.35.4.357

Gardner, R. A. (1998, October 12). Recommendations for Dealing with Parents
who Induce a Parental Alienation Syndrome in their Children. *Journal
of Divorce & Remarriage, 28*(3-4), 1-23. doi:https://doi.org/10.1300/
J087v28n03_01

Gardner, R. A. (1998). *The parental alienation syndrome: A guide for mental
health and legal professionals* (2nd ed.). Cresskill, NJ, USA: Creative
Therapeutics.

Gelinas, D. J. (1983). The persisting negative effects of incest. *Psychiatry:
Journal for the Study of Interpersonal Processes, 46*(4), 312-332. Retrieved
January 17, 2021, from https://psycnet.apa.org/record/1984-20729-001

Gentner, M. B., & O'Connor-Leppert, M. L. (2019). Environmental influences on health and development: nutrition, substance exposure, and adverse childhood experiences. *Developmental Medicine & Child Neurology, 61*(9), 989-1116. doi:https://doi.org/10.1111/dmcn.14149

Gerba, C. P. (2019). *Environmental and Pollution Science* (3 ed.). (M. L. Brusseau, I. L. Pepper, & C. P. Gerba, Eds.) Tucson, Arizona, America: Academic Press. doi:https://doi.org/10.1016/C2017-0-00480-9

Gerhardt, C. (2019). *Families in Motion: Dynamics in Diverse Contexts.* (S. University, Ed.) Birmingham, Alabama, USA: SAGE Publications, Inc.

Giancarlo, C. (2019). *Parentectomy.* Victoria, BC, Canada: Tell Well Talent.

Giorgi, A. (2009). *The Descriptive Phenomenological Method in Psychology: A Modified Husserlian Approach.* Duquesne University Press.

Giorgi, A. (2009). *The descriptive phenomenological method in psychology; a modified Husserlian approach.* Pittsburgh, USA: Duquesne Press.

Given, L. M. (2008). *Lived Experience* (Vols. 1-0). Thousand Oaks, California, America: The SAGE Encyclopedia of Qualitative Research Methods. doi:https://dx-doi-org.ezproxy.usc.edu.au/10.4135/9781412963909.n250

Godbout, E., & Parent, C. (2012, January 23rd). The Life Paths and Lived Experiences of Adults Who Have Experienced Parental Alienation: A Retrospective Study. *Journal of Divorce & Remarriage, 53*(1), 34-54. doi:https://doi-org.ezproxy.usc.edu.au/10.1080/10502556.2012.635967

Godin, K., Stapleton, J., Kirkpatrick, S. I., Hanning, R. M., & Leatherdale, S. T. (2015, October 22). Applying systematic review search methods to the grey literature: a case study examining guidelines for school-based breakfast programs in Canada. *Systematic Reviews, 4*(138), 27. doi:https://doi.org/10.1186/s13643-015-0125-0

Goldin, D. S., & Salani, D. (2020, May). Parental Alienation Syndrome: What Health Care Providers Need to Know. *The Journal for Nurse Practitioners, 16*(5), 344-348. doi:https://doi.org/10.1016/j.nurpra.2020.02.006

Gomez, A., Chinchilla, J., Vazquez, A., Lopez-Rodriguez, L., Paredes, B., & Martinez, M. (2020, April 23). Recent advances, misconceptions, untested assumptions, and future research agenda for identity fusion theory. *Social and Personality Psychology Compass, 14*(6), 1-24. doi:https://doi-org.ezproxy.usc.edu.au/10.1111/spc3.12531

Goodman, R. (2017). Contemporary Trauma Theory and Trauma-Informed Care in Substance Use Disorders: A Conceptual Model for Integrating Coping and Resilience. *Advances in Social Work, 18*(1), 186-201. doi:10.18060/21312

Green, J. G., McLaughlin, K. A., Berglund, P. A., Gruber, M. J., Sampson, N. A., Zaslavsky, A. M., & Kessler, R. C. (2010). Childhood adversities and adult psychiatric disorders in the National Comorbidity Survey Replication I: Associations with first onset of DSM-IV disorders. *Archives of General Psychiatry, 67*(2), 113-123. doi:https://doi-org.ezproxy.usc.edu.au/10.1001/archgenpsychiatry.2009.186

Gye, B. (2023, May 3). CEO Community Mental Health Australia. (A. M. Price-Tobler, Interviewer) NSW, Australia.

Haines, J., Matthewson, M., & Turnbull, M. (2020). *Understanding and Managing Parental Alienation. A Guide to Assessment and Intervention.* (Vol. 1). Abingdon, Oxon, England: Routledge. Retrieved October 31, 2020

Hamilton, J. C., & Kouchi, K. A. (2018, January 5). Factitious Disorders and the Adjudication of Claims of Physical and Mental Injury. *Psychological Injury and Law*(N/A), 9-21. doi:https://doi-org.ezproxy.usc.edu.au/10.1007/s12207-017-9310-x

Harman, J. (2016). 'Parental alienation': What it means and why it matters. *The Conversation*, 1-5. Retrieved January 16, 2021, from https://theconversation.com/parental-alienation-what-it-means-and-why-it-matters-60763

Harman, J. J., Leder-Elder, S., & Biringen, Z. (2019). Prevalence of adults who are the targets of parental alienating behaviors and their impact. *Children and Youth Services Review, 106*, 1-21. doi:doi.org/10.1016/j.childyouth.2019.104471

Harman, J. J., Matthewson, M. L., & Baker, A. J. (2021, May 10). Losses Experienced by Children Alienated from a Parent. *Current Opinion in Psychology*, 1-21. doi:https://doi.org/10.1016/j.copsyc.2021.05.002

Harper, D. (2008). *Reflexivity: A Practical Guide for Researchers in Health and Social Sciences.* Oxford.

Harris, C. H. (2008). Intimate partner homicide and familicide in Western Australia. *International conference on homicide.* Retrieved May 28, 2023, from https://usc.primo.exlibrisgroup.com/discovery/fulldisplay?docid=cdi_rmit_indexes_9781921532429er_homicide_and_familicide_ in_Western_Au_62207_CINCH_Health&context=PC&vid=61USC_INST:61USC&lang=en&search_scope=CentralIndex&adaptor=Primo%20Central&tab=Central

Henderson, A. (2018). *Enid Lyons. Leading Lady to a Nation* (2 ed.). Redlands Bay, Qld, Australia: Jeparit Press.

Herman, J. (1992). Complex PTSD: A syndrome in survivors of prolonged and repeated trauma. *Journal of Traumatic Stress, 5*(3), 377-391. doi:10.1002/jts.2490050305

Herman, J. L. (2002, January 4). Recovery from psychological trauma. *Psychiatry and Clinical Neurosciences, 52*(1), S98-S103. doi:https://doi-org.ezproxy.usc.edu.au/10.1046/j.1440-1819.1998.0520s5S145.x

Hertz, R. (1997). *Reflexivity and Voice.* SAGE Publications Inc.

Hesse-Bibber, S. N., & Piatelli, D. (2012). *The Feminist Practice of Holistic Reflexivity.* Sage Publications Inc. doi:https://doi.org/10.4135/9781483384740

Hetherington, M. E. (1993). An overview of the Virginia Longitudinal Study of Divorce and Remarriage with a focus on early adolescence. *Journal of Family Psychology, 7*(1), 39-56. doi:http://dx.doi.org.ezproxy.usc.edu.au:2048/10.1037/0893-3200.7.1.39

Hickey, S., & Nedim, U. (2020, August 25). *Abducting Your Own Child Can Amount to a Crime in Australia.* Retrieved June 19, 2021, from Sydney Criminal Lawyers: https://www.mondaq.com/australia/crime/979016/abducting-your-own-child-can-amount-to-a-crime-in-australia

Horsfall, D., & Pinn, J. (2009). Writing collaboratively. In S. Grace (Ed.). The Netherlands: Sense Publishers. Retrieved November 5, 2022, from https://researchdirect.westernsydney.edu.au/islandora/object/uws%3A25977

Hughes, A. E., Crowell, S. E., Uyeji, L., & Coan, J. A. (2012, January). A Developmental Neuroscience of Borderline Pathology: Emotion Dysregulation and Social Baseline Theory. *Journal of Abnormal Child Psychology, 40*(1), 21-33. doi:10.1007/s10802-011-9555-x

ISNAF. (2021). *Parental Alienation Glossary of Terms.* Retrieved January 16, 2021, from The International Support Network of Alienated Families: https://isnaf.info/parental-alienation-glossary-of-terms/

Jaber, N. (2021, January 14). *NIH National Cancer Institute.* Retrieved June 30, 2023, from Study Suggests a Link Between Stress and Cancer Coming Back:

https://www.cancer.gov/news-events/cancer-currents-blog/2021/cancer-returning-stress-hormones

Jaffe, P. G., Campbell, M., Hamilton, L. H., & Juodis, M. (2012). Children in Danger of Domestic Homicide. *Chile Abuse & Neglect, 36*(1), 71-74. doi:-doi: 10.1016/j.chiabu.2011.06.008

Jaffe, P., Dawson, M., & Campbell, M. (2013). Canadian perspectives on preventing domestic homicides: Developing a national collaborative approach to domestic homicide review committees. *Canadian Journal of Criminology and Criminal Justice Policy, 55*(1), 137-155. doi:Doi: 10.3138/cjccj.2011.E.53

Johnson, C. H. (2005). *Come with Daddy: Child Murder-Suicide After Family Breakdown.* Crawley, W.A: The University of Western Australia Publishing. doi:DOI: 10.3316/informit.1920694420

Johnson, C.H. (2008). Intimate partner homicide and familicide in Western Australia. *International conference on homicide.* Australian Criminology Database. Retrieved May 28, 2023, from https://usc.primo.exlibrisgroup.com/discovery/fulldisplay?docid=cdi_rmit_indexes_9781921532429er_homicide_and_familicide_in_Western_Au_62207_CINCH_Health&context=PC&vid=61USC_INST:61USC&lang=en&search_scope=CentralIndex&adaptor=Primo%20Central&tab=Central

Johnson, C. H. (2009). "Intimate Partner Homicide, Familicide and Child Trauma and the Need for. (pp. 1-9). Curtin University of Technology. Retrieved May 28, 2023, from https://aija.org.au/wp-content/uploads/2017/11/Johnson1.pdf

Jones, E. (1991). *Working with Adult Survivors of Child Sexual Abuse.* London, England: Routledge.

Judd, F., Jackson, H., Fraser, C., Murray, G., Robins, G., & Komiti, A. (2006). Understanding suicide in Australian farmers. *Social Psychiatry and Psychiatric Epidemiology, 41*(1), 1-10. doi:https://doi.org/10.1007/s00127-005-0007-1

Karlsson, L. C., Antfolk, J., Putkonen, H., Amon, S., Guerreiro, J. d., De Vogel, V., . . . Weizmann-Henelius, G. (2021). Familicide: A Systematic Literature Review. *TRAUMA, VIOLENCE, & ABUSE, 22*(1), 83-98. doi:https://doi.org/10.1177/1524838018821955

Kelly, J. B. (2010). Commentary on "family bridges: using insights from social science to reconnect parents and alienation children" (Warshak, 2010). *Family Court Review, 48*(1), 81-90. doi:https://doi.org/10.1111/j.1744-1617.2009.01289.x

Kessler, R. R. (2000). Posttraumatic stress disorder: The burden to the individual and to society. *The Journal of Clinical Psychiatry, 61*(5), 4-14. Retrieved August 28, 2021, from https://psycnet-apa-org.ezproxy.usc.edu.au/record/2000-15312-001

Kilpatrick, D. G., Ruggiero, K. J., Acierno, R., Saunders, B. E., Resnick, H. S., & Best, C. (2003). Violence and risk of PTSD, major depression, substance abuse/dependence, and comorbidity: Results from the National Survey of Adolescents. *Journal of Consulting and Clinical Psychology, 71*(4), 692-700. doi:https://doi.org/10.1037/0022-006X.71.4.692

King, N. (2004). *Using Interviews in Qualitative Research.* London: SAGE Publications Ltd.

Kirkwood, D. (2012). *'Just say goodbye': parents who kill their children in the context of separation.* Discussion paper, Domestic Violence Resource Centre, Victoria, Collingwood. Retrieved May 28, 2023, from https://vgls.sdp.sirsidynix.net.au/client/search/asset/1288903

Kleinsorge, C., & Covitz, L. M. (2012, April). Impact of Divorce on Children: Developmental Considerations. *Pediatrics in Review*, 147-155. doi:https://doi.org/10.1542/pir.33-4-147

Korosi, S. (2017, November 4). *Overcoming Parental Alienation.* Retrieved January 11, 2022, from Dialogue in Growth: https://dialogueingrowth.com.au/parental-alienationevidence-based-reunification-available-in-australia/

Kotze, D. (2020, January 30). F W de Klerk made a speech 31 years ago that ended apartheid: why he did it. *The Conversation*, 1-4. Retrieved December 4, 2022, from https://theconversation.com/fw-de-klerk-made-a-speech-31-years-ago-that-ended-apartheid-why-he-did-it-130803

Kruk, E. (2022). *Strategies to reunite alienated parents and their children.* Retrieved January 11, 2022, from Child Rights NGO: https://childrightsngo.com/parent-child-reunification-after-alienation/

Larsson, S. C., Carter, P., Kar, S., Vithayathil, M., Mason, A. M., Michaelsson, K., & Burgess, S. (2020, July 23). Smoking, alcohol consumption, and cancer: A mendelian randomisation study in UK Biobank and international genetic consortia participants. *PLoS Medicine, 17*(7). doi:doi: 10.1371/journal.pmed.1003178

Lauterbach, A. A. (2018, November). Hermeneutic Phenomenological Interviewing: Going Beyond Semi-Structured Formats to Help Participants Revisit Experience. *The Qualitative Report, 23*(11), 2882-2898. Retrieved July 10, 2021, from https://www-proquest-com.ezproxy.usc.edu.au/docview/2155621343?pq-origsite=primo&accountid=28745

Lee-Maturana, S., Matthewson, M. L., & Dwan, C. (2020, May 18). Targeted Parents Surviving Parental Alienation: Consequences of the Alienation and Coping Strategies. *Journal of Child and Family Studies, 29*, 1-49. doi:https://doi-org.ezproxy.usc.edu.au/10.1007/s10826-020-01725-1

Lewis, C. F., & Bunce, S. C. (2003, December). Filicidal mothers and the impact of psychosis on maternal filicide. *The Journal of the American Academy of Psychiatry and the Law, 31*(4), 459-470. Retrieved 28 5, 2023, from https://jaapl.org/content/31/4/459

Lewis, D. (2003). Voices in the social construction of bullying at work: exploring multiple realities in further and higher education. *International Journal of Decision Making, 4*(1), 65-81. Retrieved December 5, 2022, from https://www.researchgate.net/publication/247831471_Voices_in_the_social_construction_of_bullying_at_work_exploring_multiple_realities_in_further_and_higher_education

Liamputtong, P. (2019). *Sensitive Research Methodology and Approach: An Introduction.* Singapore: Springer Nature. doi:https://doi.org/10.1007/978-981-10-5251-4_122

Liebrucks, A. (2001, June). The Concept of Social Construction. *Theoretical psychology, 11*(3), 363-391. doi:https://doi-org.ezproxy.usc.edu.au/10.1177/0959354301113005

Linabary, J. R., Corple, D. J., & Cooky, C. (2020, August 29). Of wine and whiteboards: Enacting feminist reflexivity in collaborative research. *Qualitative Research, 21*(5), 719-735. doi:https://doi-org.ezproxy.usc.edu.au/10.1177/1468794120946988

Liu, S., Yang, H., Cheng, M., & Miao, T. (2022, August 7). Family Dysfunction and Cyberchondria among Chinese Adolescents: A Moderated Mediation Model. *International Journal of Environmental Research and Public Health, 19*(15), 1-23. doi: doi: 10.3390/ijerph19159716

Lo, I. (2019, December 12). *Did You Have to Grow Up Too Soon?* Retrieved June 16, 2021, from Psychology Today: https://www.psychologytoday.com/au/blog/living-emotional-intensity/201912/did-you-have-grow-too-soon

Locke, E. (2001). Motivation, Cognition, and Action: An Analysis of Studies of Task Goals and Knowledge. *Applied Psychology, 49*(3), 408-429. doi: https://doi-org.ezproxy.usc.edu.au/10.1111/1464-0597.00023

Lorandos, D., & Bernet, W. (2020). *Parental Alienation Science and Law.* Springfield, Illinois, America: Charles C Thomas. Retrieved November 6, 2020

Lorandos, D., Bernet, W., & Sauber, S. R. (2013). *Overview of Parental Alienation, in Parental Alienation: The Handbook for Mental Health and Legal Professionals.* (B. a. Lorandos, Ed.) Springfield, Illinois, America: Charles C Thomas.

Mahmood, K. (2006). Dr. Elisabeth Kubler-Ross stages of dying and phenomenology of grief. *Annals of King Edward Medical University, 12*(2), 232-233. doi:DOI: https://doi.org/10.21649/akemu.v12i2.882

Martin, J., & Pritchard, R. (2010). *Learning from tragedy : homicide within families in New Zealand 2002-2006.* Retrieved May 28 2023, from New Zealand Family Violence Clearinghouse: https://library.nzfvc.org.nz/cgi-bin/koha/opac-detail.pl?biblionumber=2490

McCann, L. I., & Pearlman, L. A. (1990, August 28). Vicarious traumatization: A framework for understanding the psychological effects of working with victims. *Journal of Traumatic Stress, 3*(1), 131-149. Retrieved August 28, 2021, from https://psycnet-apa-org.ezproxy.usc.edu.au/record/1990-17844-001

McCarty, D. E. (2020, March 22). Parental Alienation: Eric Carroll--Dad Talk Today host--flips the questions back to Dawn and Alyse. *Dad Talk Today.* (E. Carroll, Interviewer, & A. Price-Tobler, Editor) Florida, America. Retrieved June 7, 7.6.2021, from https://humanlypossiblechannel.com/humanly-possible-videos

McGowan, A. (2021, July 24). Radicalism mixed with openness: how Desmond Tutu used his gifts to help end Apartheid. *The Conversation*, 1-5. Retrieved December 4, 2022, from https://theconversation.com/radicalism-mixed-with-openness-how-desmond-tutu-used-his-gifts-to-help-end-apartheid-156499

McLaughlin, K. A., Green, J. G., Berglund, P. A., Gruber, M. J., Sampson, N. A., Zaslavsky, A. M., & Kessler, R. C. (2010). Childhood adversities and adult psychiatric disorders in the National Comorbidity Survey Replication I: Associations with first onset of DSM-IV disorders. *Archives of General Psychiatry, 67*(2), 113-123. doi: https://doi-org.ezproxy.usc. edu.au/10.1001/archgenpsychiatry.2009.186

McWhorter, M. R. (2019, August 13). Balancing Value Bracketing with the Integration of Moral Values in Psychotherapy: Evaluation of a Clinical Practice from the Perspective of Catholic Moral Theology. *The Linacre Quarterly, 86*(2-3), 207-224. doi:doi: 10.1177/0024363919856810

Mead, G. H. (1934). *MIND, SELF, and SOCIETY from the standpoint of a social behaviorist.* Chicago, United States: The University of Chicago Press.

Meland, E., Furuholmen, D., & Jahanlu, D. (2023, April 23). Parental alienation – a valid experience? *Scandinavian Journal of Public Health, 0*(0), 1-14. doi:https://doi.org/10.1177/14034948231168978

Merriam, S. B., & Tisdell, E. J. (2016). *Qualitative research: A guide to design and implementation* (4 ed.). San Francisco, America: Newark-Wiley.

Metzler, M., Merrick, M. T., Klevens, J., Ports, K. A., & Ford, D. C. (2017). Adverse childhood experiences and life opportunities: Shifting the narrative. *Children and Youth Services Review, 72*, 141-149. doi:https://doi. org/10.1016/j.childyouth.2016.10.021

Michalchuk, S., & Martin, S. L. (2019). Vicarious Resilience and Growth in Psychologists Who Work With Trauma Survivors: An Interpretive Phenomenological Analysis. *Professional Psychology: Research and Practice, 50*(3), 145-154. doi:http://dx.doi.org.ezproxy.usc.edu.au:2048/ 10.1037/pro0000212

Milloy, J. (2010). Attending to the somatic fringes of the moment (panel presentation). *International Human Science Research Conference.* Seattle.

Montagna, P. (2019). Parental alienation and parental alienation syndrome. In *Psychoanalysis, Law, and Society* (pp. 188-200). Routledge. doi:10.4324/ 9780429202438

Moon, K., & Blackman, D. (2017, May 2). *A guide to ontology, epistemology, and philosophical perspectives for interdisciplinary researchers.* Retrieved May 13, 2023, from Integration and Implementation Insights: https://i2insights. org/2017/05/02/philosophy-for-interdisciplinarity/#:~:text=and%20

Blackman%202014)-,Ontology,of%20objects%20they%20are%20 researching.

Morgan, A., Ahmad, N., & Webster, M. (2020). *The Clinical and Legal Management of Parental Alienation in the United Kingdom.* Final Report, University of Wolver Hampton. Retrieved January 13, 2022, from https:// pasg.info/app/uploads/2021/03/Morgan-et-al.-2020-PA-in-UK.pdf

Mouzos, J., & Rushforth, C. (2003). Family homicide in Australia. *Trends & issues in Crime and Criminal Justice*(255), 1-6. Retrieved May 28, 2023, from https://www.aic.gov.au/publications/tandi/tandi255

Muris, P., Merckelbach, H., de Jong, P. J., & Ollendick, T. H. (2002, February). The etiology of specific fears and phobias in children: a critique of the non-associative account. *Behaviour Research and Therapy, 40*(2), 185-195. doi:https://doi.org/10.1016/S0005-7967(01)00051-1

National Library of Medicine. (2003). Chapter 3 The Core Competencies Needed for Health Care Professionals. In *Health Professions Education* (pp. 1-25). Bethesda, MD, USA. Retrieved December 4, 2022, from https://www. ncbi.nlm.nih.gov/books/NBK221519/

National School of Healthcare Science. (n.d.). *Understanding different types of bias.* Retrieved May 14, 2023, from NHS England: https://nshcs. hee.nhs.uk/about/equality-diversity-and-inclusion/conscious-inclusion/ understanding-different-types-of-bias/

Natoli, A. P., Paez, M. M., & McGowan, T. (2022, June 17). Psychodynamic psychotherapy. *Reference Module in Neuroscience and Biobehavioural Psychology.* doi:https://doi.org/10.1016/B978-0-323-91497-0.00074-6

Nesvig, K. (2022, February 3). *The Simple, 5-Minute Habits That Therapists Say Will Reduce WFH Burnout.* Retrieved December 5, 2022, from Apartment Therapy: https://www.apartmenttherapy.com/habits-reduce-work-from-home-burnout-37032803

Newby, J. M., & McElroy, E. (2020, January). The impact of internet-delivered cognitive behavioural therapy for health anxiety on cyberchondria. *Journal of Anxiety Disorders, 69*, 1-8. doi:https://doi.org/10.1016/j. janxdis.2019.102150

Nowell, L. S., Norris, J. M., White, D. E., & Moules, N. J. (2017, October 2). Thematic Analysis: Striving to Meet the Trustworthiness Criteria. *International Journal of Qualitative Methods, 16*(1), 1-13. doi:10.1177/ 1609406917733847

NSW Government Health. (2020, January 20). *What is a person-centred approach?* Retrieved February 16, 2021, from NSW Government Health: https://www.health.nsw.gov.au/mentalhealth/psychosocial/principles/Pages/person-centred.aspx

Office of Juvenile Justice and Delinquency Prevention. (2010). *The Crime of Family Abduction. A Child's and Parent's Perspective.* Washington , D.C, America: U.S Department of Justice. Retrieved June 19, 2021, from https://www.ojp.gov/pdffiles1/ojjdp/229933.pdf?fbclid=IwAR3lr7mc-C6eC3vCgzpT6Z8rbt70i9r7ou0pSZJHMBkopGP6cs9UgLyKfuL0

One Door Mental Health. (2020, June). *Join Our Board.* Retrieved August 17, 2023, from One Door Mental Health: https://www.onedoor.org.au/news-updates/enews/enews-june-2020/join-our-board

Opperman, J. (2004, July-August). Parental Alienation Syndrome: what do you do when your child stops seeing you as mom or dad? *Children's Voice, 13*(4), 23-25. Retrieved August 14, 2021, from https://www-proquest-com.ezproxy.usc.edu.au/docview/203947284?accountid=28745

Pang, B. (2019). *Handbook of Research Methods in Health Social Sciences Ethnographic Method.* (P. Liamputtong, Ed.) Singapore: Springer Nature. doi:https://doi.org/10.1007/978-981-10-5251-4_81

Parental Alienation Study Group. (2022). *PASG info.* Retrieved February 28, 2022, from Parental Alienation Study Group: https://pasg.info/

Peavey, F. (1990). *Strategic Questioning Manual: A Powerful Tool for Personal and Social Change.* Retrieved July 10, 2021, from The Commons Social Change Library: https://commonslibrary.org/strategic-questioning/

Perry, B. D. (2003). *Effects of Traumatic Events on Children.* Retrieved July 20, 2021, from Child Trauma Academy. A Learning Community: http://fa-sett.no/filer/perry-handout-effects-of-trauma.pdf

Perry, B. D. (2021). *ChildTrauma Academy History.* Retrieved July 20, 2021, from ChildTrauma Academy: https://7079168e-705a-4dc7-be05-2218087aa989.filesusr.com/ugd/aa51c7_237459a7e16b4b7e9d2c-4837c908eefe.pdf

Peterson, A. J., Joseph, J., Feit, M., Medicine, I., & Council, N. (2014). *New Directions in Child Abuse and Neglect Research.* National Academies Press. doi:DOI:10.17226/18331

Pham, M. T., Rajic, A., Greig, J. D., Sargeant, J. M., Papadopoulos, A., & McEwen, S. A. (2014, July 24). Wiley Research Synthesis Methods. *PMC*

US National Library of Medicine National Institutes of Health, 5(4), 371-385. doi:10.1002/jrsm.1123

Pier, K. S., Marin, L. K., Wilsnack, J., & Goodman, M. (2016, April 1). The Neurobiology of Borderline Personality Disorder. *Psychiatric Times, 33*(3), 1-7. Retrieved June 7, 2021, from Psychiatric Times: https://www.psychiatrictimes.com/view/neurobiology-borderline-personality-disorder

Price-Tobler, A., & McCarty, D. E. (2021, September 1st). Adult Survivors of Severe PA: Working Toward a New Solution to End PA. *Contemporary Family Magazine*(3), pp. 38-39. doi:https://www.flipsnack.com/contemporaryfamily/complimentary-contemporary-family-magazine-fall-2021/full-view.html

Putkonen, H., Eronon, M., Almiron, M., Cederwall, J., & Weizmann-Henelius, G. (2011). Gender Differences in Filicide Offense Characteristics-A Comprehensive Register Based Study of Child Murder in Two European Countries. *Child abuse and neglect, 35*(5), 319-328. doi:doi: 10.1016/j.chiabu.2011.01.007

Raheim, M., Magnussen, L. H., Sekse, R. J., Lunde, A., Jacobsen, T., & Blystad, A. (2016, June 14). Researcher–researched relationship in qualitative research: Shifts in positions and researcher vulnerability. *International Journal of Qualitative Studies in Health and Well-being, 11*. doi:doi: 10.3402/qhw.v11.30996

Rand, D. C. (1997, December 16). The Spectrum of Parental Alienation Syndrome (PART II). *American Journal of Forensic Psychology, 15*(4), 1. Retrieved March 20, 2020, from https://canadiancrc.com/Parental_Alienation_Syndrome_Canada/randp2.pdf

Reinharz, S. (1992). *Feminist methods in social research.* New York: Oxford University Press.

Resnick, P. J. (1969, September). Child Murder by Parents: A Psychiatric Review of Filicide. *The American Journal of Psychiatry, 126*(3), 352-334. doi:https://doi.org/10.1176/ajp.126.3.325

Roberts, R. (2020, June 6). Humanly Possible Channel. (D. McCarty, & A. M. Price-Tobler, Interviewers) Retrieved June 10, 2021, from https://www.youtube.com/watch?v=CX7cBkAbzgU

Rosenberg, M. B. (2015). *Nonviolent Communication: A Language of Life* (3 ed.). (L. Leu, Ed.) Encinitas, California, USA: PuddleDancer Press.

Ross, D. (2020). *The Revolutionary Social Worker. The Love Ethic Model.* Brisbane, Australia: Revolutionaries.

Ruggles, S. (1994, February). The Origins of African-American Family Structure. *American Sociological Review, 59*(1), 1-17. doi:10.2307/2096137

Saini, S. M., Hoffman, C. R., Pantelis, C., Everall, I. P., & Bousman, C. A. (2019, February). Systematic review and critical appraisal of child abuse measurement instruments. *Psychiatry Research, 272*, 106-113. doi:10.1016/j.psychres.2018.12.068

Salkind, N. (1991). *Exploring research* (3 ed.). (P. Janzow, Ed.) New Jersey: Simon & Schuster. Retrieved June 28, 2016

Saunders, B., Sim, J., Kingstone, T., Baker, S., Waterfield, J., Bartlam, B., . . . Jinks, C. (2017, September 14). Saturation in qualitative research: exploring its conceptualization and operationalization. *Quality and Quantity, 52*(4), 1893-1907. doi:doi: 10.1007/s11135-017-0574-8

Schore, A. N. (2002). Dysregulation of the right brain: a fundamental mechanism of traumatic attachment and the psychopathogenesis of posttraumatic stress disorder. *Australian and New Zealand Journal of Psychiatry, 36*(1), 9-30. Retrieved June 7, 2021, from http://eds.b.ebscohost.com.ezproxy.usc.edu.au:2048/eds/pdfviewer/pdfviewer?vid=0&sid=4a2bbe-fb-d70a-4498-853f-f8d627561593%40sessionmgr103

Schore, A. N. (2002). Dysregulation of the right brain: a fundamental mechanism of traumatic attachment and the psychopathogenesis of posttraumatic stress disorder. *Australian and New Zealand Journal of Psychiatry, 36*(1), 9-30. doi:10.1046/j.1440-1614.2002.00996.x.

Schore, A. N. (2009, April 1). *Relational Trauma and the Developing Right Brain. An Interface of Psychoanalytic Self Psychology and Neuroscience.* doi:10.1111/j.1749-6632.2009.04474.x

Schultheiss, D. E., & Wallace, E. (2012). *An introduction to social constructionism in vocational psychology and career development* (Vol. 4). Brill. Retrieved March 31, 2023, from https://ebookcentral.proquest.com/lib/usc/detail.action?docID=3034785#

Scott, P. D. (1973, April). Parents who kill their Children. *HeinOnline, 13*(2), 120-126. Retrieved May 28, 2023, from https://heinonline-org.ezproxy.usc.edu.au/HOL/Page?collection=journals&handle=hein.journals/mdsclw13&id=125&men_tab=srchresults

Sher, L. (2017). Parental alienation: the impact on men's mental health. *International Journal of Adolescent Medicine and Health; Berlin, 29*(3), 1-5. doi:10.1515/ijamh-2015-0083

Shivayogi, P. (2013). Vulnerable population and methods for their safeguard. *Perspectives in Clinical Research, 4*(1), 53-57. doi:10.4103/2229-3485.106389

Silva, E., Till, A., & Adshead, G. (2018, January 2). Ethical dilemmas in psychiatry: When teams disagree. *Cambridge University Press, 23*(4), 231-239. doi:10.1192/apt.bp.116.016147

Silverman, D. (1997). *Validity and credibility in qualitative research. The alternative paradigm.* (G. Miller, & R. Dingwall, Eds.) London: Sage.

Sorsoli, L., Kia-Keating, M., Grossman, F. K., & Mallinckrodt, B. (2008). "I Keep That Hush-Hush": Male Survivors of Sexual Abuse and the Challenges of Disclosure. *Journal of counselling psychology, 55*(3), 333-345. doi:10.1037/0022-0167.55.3.333

Starcevic, V. (2017, May). Cyberchondria: Challenges of Problematic Online Searches for Health-Related Information. *Psychotherapy and Psychosomatics, 86*(3), 129-133. doi:https://doi.org/10.1159/000465525

Stein, A. (2021). *Terror, Love and Brainwashing* (2 ed.). New York, United States of America: Routledge.

Strang, H. (1996, March 1). *Children as victims of homicide.* Retrieved May 28, 2023, from Australian Government. Australian Institute of Criminology: https://www.aic.gov.au/publications/tandi/tandi53

Stroud, J. (2008, November 1). A psychosocial analysis of child homicide. *Critical Social Policy, 28*(4), 482-505. doi:https://doi-org.ezproxy.usc.edu.au/10.1177/0261018308095281

Sullivan, M. J., Ward, P. A., & Deutsch, R. M. (2010, January). OVERCOMING BARRIERS FAMILY CAMP: A PROGRAM FOR HIGH-CONFLICT DIVORCED FAMILIES WHERE A CHILD IS RESISTING CONTACT WITH A PARENT. *Family Court Review, 48*(1), 116-135. doi:10.1111/j.1744-1617.2009.01293.x

Taylor, K. (2017). *Brain Washing. The Science of Thought Control* (2 ed.). Oxford, United Kingdom, England: Oxford Landmark Science.

Teicher, M. H., & Samson, J. A. (2013, October 1). Childhood Maltreatment and Psychopathology: A Case for Ecophenotypic Variants as Clinically and

Neurobiologically Distinct Subtypes. *The American Journal of Psychiatry*. doi:https://doi-org.ezproxy.usc.edu.au/10.1176/appi.ajp.2013.12070957

Teicher, M. H., & Samson, J. A. (2013, October 1). Childhood Maltreatment and Psychopathology: A Case for Ecophenotypic Variants as Clinically and Neurobiologically Distinct Subtypes. *The American Journal of Psychiatry*. doi:10.1176/appi.ajp.2013.12070957

Templer, K., Matthewson, M., Haines, J., & Cox, G. (2016, October 3). Recommendations for best practice in response to parental alienation: findings from a systematic review. *Journal of Family Therapy, 39*(1), 103-122. doi:10.1111/1467-6427.12137

The ATLEN. (2017, November 26). *Aotearoa Therapists with Lived Experience Network*. Retrieved November 14, 2022, from The ATLEN: https://theatlen.wordpress.com/2017/11/26/therapist-with-lived-experience/

Thomas, J. R., & Hognas, R. S. (2015). The Effect of Parental Divorce on the Health of Adult Children. *Longitudinal and Life Course Studies, 6*(3), 279-302. doi:10.14301/llcs.v6i3.267

Time to Put Kids First. (2019). *Home*. Retrieved 2021, from https://www.timetoputkidsfirst.org/: https://www.timetoputkidsfirst.org/

Turkat, I. D. (2000, July-September). Custody Battle Burnout. *American Journal of Family Therapy, 28*(3), 201-215. doi:10.1080/01926180050081649

University of the Health Sciences. (2021). *The Impact of Kidnapping, Shooting and Torture on Children*. Retrieved June 22, 2021, from The Center for the Study of Traumatic Stress (CSTS): https://www.cstsonline.org/resources/resource-master-list/the-impact-of-kidnapping-shooting-and-torture-on-children

van der Kolk, B. (2014). *The Body Keeps The Score* (Vol. 1). USA: Viking Penguin. Retrieved January 9 2023

Van Hoy, A., & Rzeszutek, M. (2022, August 15). Burnout and Psychological Wellbeing Among Psychotherapists: A Systematic Review. *Frontiers in Psychology*, 1-33. doi:10.3389/fpsyg.2022.928191

van Manen, M. (1990). *Researching Lived Experience : Human Science for an Action Sensitive Pedagogy*. Albany, New York, USA: State University of New York Press.

Verrocchio, M. C., Baker, A. J., & Bernet, W. (2016, February 16). Associations between Exposure to Alienating Behaviors, Anxiety, and Depression in an

Italian Sample of Adults. *Journal of Forensic Sciences, 61*(3), 692-698. doi:10.1111/1556-4029.13046

Verrocchio, M. C., Marchetti, D., Carrozzino, D., Compare, D., & Fulcheri, M. (2019). Depression and quality of life in adults perceiving exposure to parental alienation behaviors. *Health and Quality of Life Outcomes, 17*(14), 1-9. doi:10.1186/s12955-019-1080-6

Viljoen, M., & van Rensburg, E. (2014, May 8). Exploring the Lived Experiences of Psychologists Working With Parental Alienation Syndrome. *Journal of Divorce & Remarriage, 55*(4), 253-275. doi:10.1080/10502556.2014.90 1833

Wallerstein, J. S. (1985). Children of Divorce: Preliminary Report of a Ten-Year Follow-up of Older Children and Adolescents. *Journal of the American Academy of Child Psychiatry, 24*(5), 545-553. doi:10.1016/ S0002-7138(09)60055-8

Walter, M. (2019). *Social Research Methods* (4 ed.). (C. Leslie, Ed.) Docklands, Victoria, Australia: Oxford University Press.

Wamsley, L. (2021, June 2). *A Guide To Gender Identity Terms*. Retrieved November 19, 2022, from National Public Radio: https://www.npr. org/2021/06/02/996319297/gender-identity-pronouns-expression-guide-lgbtq#gender

Warshak, R. A. (2013). *What is Parental Alienation*. Retrieved June 26, 2021, from Dr Richard A Warshak: https://www.warshak.com/publications/ what-is-parental-alienation.html

Wilcox, W. B. (2009). The Evolution of Divorce. *National Affairs*, 1-23. Retrieved July 26, 2021, from https://www.nationalaffairs.com/publi-cations/detail/the-evolution-of-divorce#:~:text=In%201969%2C%20 Governor%20Ronald,first%20no%2Dfault%20divorce%20bill.

Wilkinson, S. (1988). The role of reflexivity in feminist psychology. *Women's Studies International Forum, 11*(5), 493-502. doi:https://doi. org/10.1016/0277-5395(88)90024-6

Willig, C. (2001). *Introducing Qualitative Research in Psychology: Adventures in Theory and Method, Volume 2*. Open University Press.

Wilson, J. P., & Thomas, R. B. (2004). Empathy in the Treatment of Trauma and PTSD. Taylor & Francis Group. Retrieved February 11, 2023, from https://ebookcentral.proquest.com/lib/usc/detail.action?docID=214864& pq-origsite=primo#

Winnicott, D. W. (1960). *The Theory of the Parent-Infant Relationship.*

Wurtz, E. T., Hansen, J., Roe, O. D., & Omland, O. (2020, February 10). Asbestos exposure and haematological malignancies: a Danish cohort study. *European Journal of Epidemiology, 35*(10), 949-960. doi:doi: 10.1007/s10654-020-00609-4

Young, D. C. (2009, February). Interpretivism and Education Law Research: A Natural Fit. *Education & Law Journal, 18*(3), 203-219. Retrieved March 12, 2023, from https://www.proquest.com/scholarly-journals/ interpretivism-education-law-research-natural-fit/docview/212959444/ se-2

Zachariadou, T., Zannetos, S., Chira, S. E., Gregoriou, S., & Pavlakis, A. (2018, September 7). Prevalence and Forms of Workplace Bullying Among Health-care Professionals in Cyprus: Greek Version of "Leymann Inventory of Psychological Terror" Instrument. *Science Direct, 9*(3), 339-346. doi:10.1016/j.shaw.2017.11.003

Zareen, Z., & Larsen, D. (2018, November). Commentary: Paradigms, Axiology, and Praxeology in Medical Education Research. *Academic Medicine. Journal of the Association of American Medical Colleges, 93*(11S), S1-S7. doi:10.1097/ACM.0000000000002384

A final note about references: Including all 35 pages of references in both volumes of the twin study PhD books is a strategic decision that benefits mental health practitioners and other researchers in several ways. Firstly, it provides readers with a comprehensive resource, eliminating the need to flip back and forth between volumes to access the reference list. This saves time and makes it easier for readers to locate specific sources. Additionally, having all references readily available enhances accessibility. It allows readers to cross-reference or delve deeper into specific topics covered in each volume without searching for the cited literature elsewhere.

Moreover, maintaining consistency across both volumes ensures the research findings and conclusions continuity. For researchers and academics, having access to the full list of references facilitates the verification of information, fostering trust and confidence in the research. Lastly, leaving the references intact in both volumes preserves the coherence and integrity of the content, as removing them from one of the books might disrupt the flow. Overall, this approach is a practical and valuable resource, enhancing the accessibility, credibility, and continuity of the research presented in twin study PhD books and post-doctoral research.

Appendices

Appendix One

ACE Study Questions

Note: These questions were not offered to any study participants. The questions are only here as a guide for MHPs to read when the study refers to 'The Ace Study'. The grammar in the original listing has not been corrected either.

1. Before your 18th birthday, did a parent or other adult in the household often or very often swear at you, insult you, put you down, or humiliate you? or Act in a way that made you afraid that you might be physically hurt?

2. Before your 18th birthday, did a parent or other adult in the household often or very often push, grab, slap, or throw something at you? or ever hit you so hard that you had marks or were injured?

3. Before your 18th birthday, did an adult or person at least five years older than you ever touch or fondle you or have you touched their body in a sexual way? Or Attempt or actually have oral, anal, or vaginal intercourse with you?

4. Did you often or very often feel that no one in your family loved you or thought you were important or special? Or Your family didn't look out for each other, feel close to each other, or support each other?

5. Did you often or very often feel that you didn't have enough to eat, had to wear dirty clothes, and had no one to protect you? Or Your parents were too drunk or high to take care of you or take you to the doctor if you needed it?

6. Were your parents ever separated or divorced?

7. Was your mother or stepmother often or very often pushed, grabbed, slapped, or had something thrown at her? or sometimes, often, or very often kicked, bitten, hit with a fist, or hit with something hard? or ever repeatedly hit over at least a few minutes or threatened with a gun or knife?

8. Did you live with anyone who was a problem drinker or alcoholic or who used street drugs?

9. Was a household member depressed or mentally ill, or did a household member attempt suicide?

10. Did a household member go to prison? (ACES Too High News, 2020, p. 1)

https://form.jotform.com/221574555560054

Appendix Two

Categories of Parental Alienation- Mild, Moderate and Severe

Please read over the following level definitions of parental alienation and see which one you identify with the most. The study is looking to recruit adult-child survivors of severe parental alienation and mental health practitioners who work with this population. If you feel that after reading these definitions, you relate to the severe category of parental alienation, please contact Alyse Price-Tobler to apply for the main study.

Mild Parental Alienation

The mild type of PAS behaviour has some degree of parental programming aimed against the TP; however, visits are not detrimentally affected, and the child can manage the transition to being around the alienated TP without too much stress (Baker, 2007). A mild level of PA is also identified when the child resisting contact with the AP starts to enjoy parenting time and relinquishes the resistance they were displaying at the start of the visit (Lorandos & Bernet, 2020).

Moderate Parental Alienation

According to Baker (2007, p. 22), the moderate type of PAS is more fearsome, and the children are described as having "some parental programming against the targeted parent" and may struggle with visitation. A moderate level of PA is identified when the child exhibits strong resistance to the suggestion of contact with their AP and is constantly oppositional toward the TP during parenting time visits. However, there are occasionally a few moments of encouraging connection between the child and the AP (Lorandos & Bernet, 2020). A further example of moderate PAS is characterised as the child being exposed to a considerable level of parental programming from the AP (Baker, 2007). This programming creates a substantial internal battle for the child when visiting an AP (Baker, 2007). In these cases, the child may have a relationship with their TP that is reasonably strong, and eventually, they settle and adapt to the visit (Baker, 2007).

Severe Parental Alienation

In cases experiencing severe levels of SPA, children are adamant in their hatred of the alienated TP, often refusing visits with them and threatening to run away if a visit is proposed (Baker, 2007). Children experiencing severe levels of PA often have an unhealthy, enmeshed alliance with the AP, sharing paranoid fantasies about the TP to the point where the child's relationship with the TP is destroyed (Baker, 2007). Friends and family may also notice that the child and AP may have an unhealthy alliance (Baker, 2007). The definition of severe parental alienation (SPA), according to Lorandos et al. (2013), involves children who persistently and adamantly refuse all contact with the TP to the extent that they may even run away or hide to avoid spending time with them. Within the SPA context, visitation may be impossible due to the children being incredibly hostile to the point where the children may become physically violent toward the supposedly hated parent (Baker, 2007).

Other ways of acting out may be present, designed to cause formidable grief to the parent visited by the alienated child (Baker, 2007). These levels can manifest in behaviours such as running away and hiding to avoid seeing the alienated parent and remaining defiant and oppositional if they are made to spend parenting time with them (Baker, 2007). In addition, some severely alienated children exhibit behaviours such as persisting in not seeing the alienated parent and stating that they do not want to partake in a relationship with them (Lorandos & Bernet, 2020, p. 550). "In many cases, the children's hostility has reached paranoid levels, that is, delusions of persecution and fears that they will be murdered in situations where there is absolutely no evidence that such will be the case" (Gardner, 2008, p. 2).

Appendix Three

Qualifying Questions for Mental Health Practitioners Who Treat Survivors of SPA

1. As a mental health practitioner, have you or are you currently treating adult survivors (not children) of severe parental alienation (SPA) instead of mild or moderate parental alienation?

2. Do you have a bachelor's degree or a post-graduate degree?

3. Would you be willing to participate in a PhD research study that explores the perspectives, practices, and experiences of mental health practitioners who treat adult survivors of child psychological abuse in the severe level of parental alienation?

✧

Appendix Four

Semi-Structured Interview Schedule (Mental Health Practitioners) Survey Questions

1. How many adult survivors of SPA have you treated?
2. How do you identify which clients are adult survivors of SPA?
3. How often do you think adult survivors of SPA are not identified and treated for something other than SPA?
4. Have you received any formal training for adult survivors of SPA? If so, where?
5. If you have not received any formal training in SPA, what have you sought out for professional development within the area of SPA?
6. What percentage of clients know they are adult survivors of SPA when they first arrive for therapy?
7. What treatment methods do you engage in when working with adult survivors of SPA?
8. Have you ever received feedback from the adult survivors of SPA about the treatment you have provided? If so, what feedback was reported?

9. How many other practitioners do you know who work with adult survivors of SPA?

10. How many other practitioners do you know who understand SPA?

11. What is your biggest concern when working with adult survivors of SPA?

12. How does working with adult survivors of SPA affect you personally, both mentally and physically?

13. What do you think needs improving regarding treatment options for adult survivors of SPA?

14. What do you think needs improving about professional development for practitioners who work with adult survivors of SPA?

15. What other programs or ideas could be developed to help other practitioners treat adult survivors of SPA?

16. What advice could you give to help other practitioners to understand the mind of an adult survivor of SPA?

17. Do you have any advice for practitioners who may wish to treat adult survivors of SPA?

18. Do you have any suggestions with regard to future treatment protocols for adult survivors of SPA?

Appendix Five

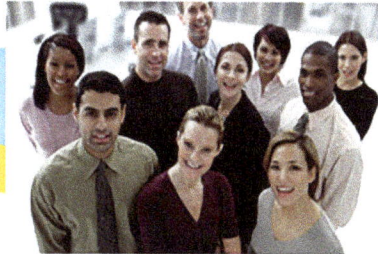

Mental Health

Practitioners...

WE NEED YOU!

Have you ever consulted an adult client
who has experienced high conflict divorce
and/or severe parental alienation
as a child or adolescent?

We are aiming to develop a greater understanding about the experiences and knowledge of mental health practitioners who have consulted with adult survivors of high conflict divorce, and or severe parental alienation (SPA).

At the moment, we believe the needs and experiences of SPA survivors are sometimes not well understood or managed by all mental health practitioners. We hope to address these issues and potentially improve support and services.

If you would like to participate, it would involve an informal interview lasting approximately 30-45 minutes. This interview is in no way evaluative. We are only interested in your opinions, experiences and views as a practitioner.

This is a great opportunity for you to contribute to furthering the education and practices of mental health practitioners, which may lead to an improvement in front line supports and services to other adult of SPA.

If you would like to participate in this study, or would like further information, then please contact the Student Researcher Alyse Price-Tobler on

email alyse.price-tobler@research.usc.edu.au and leave a contact number (if in Australia) and a convenient time to be contacted.

Please note, Privacy and confidentiality is strictly adhered to in accordance with ethical guidelines. Thankyou.

Appendix Six

Human Research Ethics Approval for Research Project

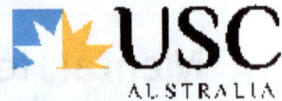

USC
AUSTRALIA

21 December 2021

A/Prof Andrew Crowden
Chair, Human Research Ethics Committee
Tel: +61 7 5430 2823
Email: humanethics@usc.edu.au

Dr Dyann Ross
Dr Peter Innes
Ms Alyse Price-Tobler
Dr Mandy Matthewson

Dear Investigators

Human research ethics approval for research project: Working with Adult Survivors of Severe Parental Alienation: Survivors and Mental Health Practitioners Perspective. A Qualitative Study (S211642)

This letter is to confirm that the USC Human Research Ethics Committee (HREC) has reviewed and granted ethics approval for this project subject to the standard conditions of approval listed below.

The period of ethics approval is from 21 December 2021 to 21 December 2024. The ethics approval number for the project is S211642. This number should be quoted on your Research Project Information Sheet and in any written communication with participants.

Ethics approval indicates that this project meets the requirements of the National Health and Medical Research Council's (NHMRC) *National Statement on Ethical Conduct in Human Research (2007)*. This does not negate the need for other approvals where relevant. It is the investigators' responsibility to ensure that all approvals relevant to this project are obtained.

If you have any queries or if you require further information, please contact us using the details above.

Yours sincerely

for
A/Prof Andrew Crowden
Chair, Human Research Ethics Committee